# The Leap Year

# The Leap Year

*One woman's desire to make sense of the rollercoaster of emotions and need for understanding after a breast cancer diagnosis and how she finds her inner strength to take on new challenges.*

## JANE DELAHAY

### accentia
*Providing professional book creation services and opportunity for independent authors to tell their story*

First published 2017

Publishing Partner: Accentia Design
Cover image: © 2017 by Anna Blatman (www.annablatman.com)
Cover design: Michelle Hessing
Copy editing: Heather Bryant

Copyright © Jane Delahay, 2017

The moral right of the author has been asserted.

All rights reserved.

Without limiting the rights under copyright restricted above, no part of this publication may be reproduced, in any form or by any means (electronic, mechanical, photocopying, recording or otherwise), without the prior written permission of both the copyright owner and the above publishing partner of this book.

Typesetting & Prepared for Publication by: Accentia Design

A Cataloguing-in-Publication record is available from the National Library of Australia.

ISBN: 978-0-6480070-6-7 (Paperback)
ISBN: 978-0-6480070-7-4 (ePub)

*For Ray*

*"When life falls apart; bend down and pick up the pieces – that's when the real magic starts"*

~ Jane Delahay

# The Leap Year

## INTRODUCTION/PREFACE

If someone had told me in the space of twelve months I would be diagnosed with breast cancer, fall in love with yoga, do a walking trek to Tuscany with nineteen other incredible women, believe in the benefits of eastern medicine, and write a book, I would have told them that they were totally delusional. It could not have been further from the life I was living.

> *"Each life has its own purpose. The ultimate goal is to achieve your destiny and enjoy life fully. Everything that happened in my life has a positive for me to take from it – even breast cancer."*
> Jane Delahay

No words have ever resonated with me more than these. It was truly a light bulb moment. I had been on this earth for forty-seven years and I truly could not think of another time that I was stopped dead in my tracks. I, along with many other people, have asked myself why. Why did I get breast cancer? What have I done to deserve this?

No one can tell you, which is possibly the hardest thing to accept when you are the 1 in 8 women who will get breast cancer in their lifetime in Australia. That is a sobering statistic, and one I had never thought about, ever.

The 22nd February, 2016 started like any other day. I still remember what I was wearing. That Monday was a gorgeous summer day and I was on my way to work. I knew I had a mammogram booked for 12.30pm, which was just routine, really; it had come about because I felt a strange, flat lump the Friday before. I had had strange lumps previously; two that were benign and taken out years ago. I didn't think it was anything different. After the tests, they sent me on my merry way; no one said a word to me.

I had barely stepped out of the radiology department when my phone rang. It was my GP, who said he needed me to come straight in. My heart was pounding, "What? Why do you want to see me?"

"We need to see you, come right away."

No explanation on the phone. I got there within fifteen minutes and sat breathlessly across the desk from my GP.

"You have breast cancer."

No one EVER wants to hear those words. But in 2016, 16,084 Australians heard that news and I was one of them. That is a truly staggering number and it is on the increase.

I grieved the disappearance of my former life. It had been taken away from me in a matter of seconds and every corner I turned around presented me with more and more anxiety. I was petrified of my life. Why was it happening to me? All I ever wanted was to be happy and healthy. Suddenly, I was neither. It was difficult and hard to accept that my life had changed forever.

I had the choice to listen to my inner self and to use my diagnosis as an opportunity to change. It was time to believe in myself.

This story is about how my life changed in an instant, how I finally found what I was supposed to do. Breast Cancer had given me the chance to start again and I had to decide what I wanted from my life.

I had the power to choose the life I desired. I could choose the plot, the cast of characters, and the movie setting; all of that and more.

We all have the ability to just be, and to do what we really desire, I needed to find that light. The challenge was so big it weighed me down, in every aspect of my being. Being diagnosed with breast cancer had changed my life so much that it became foreign to me. I was hurt, I was angry, and I felt cut off from reality.

But I found my way through the toughest road in my life. I found solace and peace in the least expected places. Encountered things and people I never knew existed. It was a profound time and opened my mind to the existence of miracles, of love, of friendship, and magic.

The life I see before me now is a stark difference to the life I had one year ago. I am a different person today; I certainly don't sweat the small stuff. I am at peace with what's happened, and I do not take my health for granted. It has been a blessing in disguise.

# CHAPTER 1

When I was first diagnosed, I told no one.

I couldn't even process it myself let alone try and to tell anyone else. I drove around my neighbourhood for a while, circling well-known streets and driving in a state of mindlessness. I stopped for a coffee and sat staring into space. It was the lead up to Easter, I remember buying a hot cross bun at the café but I couldn't eat it – my stomach was churning – so I asked if I could take it home. As soon as I sat down in the comfy velvet chair near the window, I started Googling, and then had to stop; I couldn't take any of it in. I was in shock, it couldn't be happening.

This isn't happening to me, kept going through my head. *They have made a mistake, they have the wrong person.*

I convinced myself I was overreacting; the small amount of Googling I had done said that the majority of breast lumps are benign, good, OK. That was me, then. I couldn't possibly have *cancer*.

I had an appointment with the surgeon that evening; he made a special time for me. It was nearly 6pm by the time I saw him and I sat there like a stunned mullet; he was drawing pictures and talking in another language as far as I was concerned. I remember thinking about a cartoon where the owner is telling his dog off and the caption above the dog's head says, 'blah, blah, blah, Rover, blah, blah.' That is exactly how I felt; he wasn't talking to me.

I left there with a whole lot of paper with hand drawings of boobs, and what looked like squiggles, arrows, and graphs. I had been there for an hour, and apart from my wallet being a lot lighter, I was none the wiser, nothing had sunk in.

As I left he said, "Lots of blue sky ahead, Jane."

All I could see was a bleak, grey, raining sky. I was in shock and all I could do was stand in the street afterwards and light a cigarette.

I drove around my neighbourhood for a bit longer before I realised I needed to go home. My husband had texted me asking if I was alright. I was supposed to be at the dentist and he thought something had gone wrong. Well, it had gone wrong, but it wasn't my teeth.

As I pulled into the driveway at home, I didn't even know how I was going to tell my husband and children. The big 'C'. Mum has cancer; how do you tell your children without frightening them? They were eleven and fourteen, at the time. I didn't even know what type of cancer I had exactly, so how could I tell them it would all be OK when I didn't even know?

What a mess, and how bloody inconvenient!

I had just emailed my friends in the UK to say we were coming to visit. I had things to do, places to be, and cancer wasn't one of them—not by a long shot.

I didn't say anything. I was the ostrich in the sand; *carry on, everything's fine.*

I didn't want to share my news, I wanted to hold it close to me. I couldn't bring myself to tell anyone.

I really struggled with the concept of, "Did I do this to myself?" I had been a smoker for twenty years—not a heavy smoker, but a smoker nonetheless. I had done it to myself, I was so ashamed and I didn't want to face: "I told you so."

I didn't cry, didn't have any emotion. I was silent and couldn't make one bit of sense of it all. I actually felt calm, almost like I was watching from the outside, like it was happening to someone else, not me. I had no sense of space, or time. I felt like I was in another world, not my world. My world was dandy, I loved my life.

I decided I would tell my husband and children only for the fact I had a mountain of tests to go to in the next few days and my surgery was booked for a weeks' time. I couldn't get away with not telling them. Game was up, I couldn't hide it.

There were tears and group hugs in the kitchen, but I kept telling my children I would be absolutely fine; they had found it early and I would have an operation and some treatment. I would be fine.

Of course, I was talking out of my arse because I had no idea. At that time, it could have been terminal and I would have been in a totally different boat. As a parent, I had to reassure them I would always be there for them. I believed that, and I wanted life to remain as normal as possible. Children process things so differently, I wish everyone could see the world through children's eyes; they have the most positive attitude.

"Oh well, Mum, you will be fine, and is it OK if I go to my friend's house tomorrow night?"

Actually, I welcomed the low fuss because it made it easier for me. I didn't want to talk about it, anyway. My children did not have the experience dictionary for this.

No one knows how they will cope with a cancer diagnosis until it happens to them. You can pretend to know, you can project about how you will feel, but none of what you think you will feel will be anywhere near the reality.

The 'what if's' are soul destroying, the 'I wish I hads' are torture in your head, and the private nightmares make you want to jump ship. The torment in your head is relentless and you can't stop yourself from repeating thoughts over and over projecting the future and scaring yourself shitless.

How did I even get there? What did I do to deserve it?

That one is the hardest—you blame yourself. You can never minimalise the impact of the shock news you have breast cancer. I had closely similar challenges in my life before where I was calm and OK; I couldn't understand why I felt so sad and so angry.

I had to work hard at trying not to over-think the next twelve months of treatment. Losing the sense of control when you enter the medical world is confusing and confronting and scary. I didn't understand it, I didn't choose it. It was a world away from my normal life. I worked hard to convince myself it was my new normal—whatever the hell that meant. It was such a massive process to confront, even when the prognosis was good. Nothing could fix what was happening to me. Dark clouds were circling.

I resisted the urge to Google everything; I started to and had to stop. It sent me crazy. There is way too much on that library in the sky with so much conflicting material, depressing stories, and generally an information overload. It was impossible to take in; I was going to send myself mad if I even contemplated using it as a basis for information. I had to trust that my new medical people knew what was best for me. God, I hoped so.

After three days of invasive—and quite frankly, terrifying—tests, scans, and biopsies, my pathology was in: Stage 2, Grade 2, triple positive (ER +, PR +, HER2+). That meant five different treatments: surgery, chemotherapy, Herceptin, radiotherapy, and hormone therapy. In typical fashion, I had to get the Full Monty of breast cancers; the one with all of the possible treatments and no short cuts for me.

The tumour was on the large side, 35mm, and it had to come out quickly because it was aggressive. Not what I wanted to hear.

That call came on a Friday night. I was drinking a glass of wine and smoking in my back garden; not conducive to taking a call about cancer and your impeding surgery, but I didn't care. I was in no state of mind. I still didn't think they were talking about me. It was still happening to someone else.

The weekend passed in a fog. Not only because by that time I was sleep deprived after seven days of worry-induced insomnia, I had absolutely no idea how I was going to cope with it. So I went with 'business as usual', which meant busying myself with the most inane and trivial things, anything to take my mind off what was going on. There was pain, fear, loathing, and anxiety all there in my brain, swirling around like smoke with no way of escaping.

The life I knew had gone in an instant and I was terrified of the life ahead. The life of the unknown, the life after a cancer diagnosis.

I had to take it day by day – just like asking *how do you eat an elephant?* One bite at a time.

I couldn't focus on next week. I had to focus on tomorrow, today, the next hour. There was no way I could even contemplate one month.

*Stay in the now*, I was telling myself, all the while my brain had other ideas. It was filling up fast with the thoughts of a mad woman; I had become a stranger in my own head.

Monday morning, surgery day. It was the 29th February: a leap year. I guess the good thing about that was I would not be able to anniverserise that day; it was enough that I would never forget the 22nd February. At least I only had to think about the surgery day every four years and by 2020, I was guessing I wouldn't be thinking about it at all.

I was born in a leap year. It seemed almost fitting that my diagnosis happened to me in another leap year.

Well, I went to work, determined to stick to my resolve of business as usual. I had to be at the hospital by 2pm, so I wasn't going to sit around in the morning lamenting it all. Distraction was the key. I had at least woken up with some sort of clarity.

I sent my emails and attended Monday morning meetings, no one was any the wiser. I put my 'Out of Office' notice on for two weeks and left. No one except my boss knew. My team thought I had gone for lunch, albeit a long one.

# CHAPTER 2

I hate hospitals. Not just a bit, a lot. I hate the smell. As soon as I get near one, I can feel the anxiety rising. I don't know why. Probably fear I suspect. Fear that the only reason I have to go is because there is something wrong with me, and I'd likely have to endure some awful procedure in a space that is barren of personality.

You are reduced to a very basic human being in hospitals; no one is different, you are not a person, just a number made to wear degrading hospital attire while imprisoned in a stark environment devoid of any comfort. It might as well be prison, since you cannot even leave. You are trapped in your own little white box nightmare.

I was late getting to the hospital. The staff were waiting for me and the breast care nurse was the first person I saw. She was very cheery in that kind of overprotective parent way and carrying a rather large pink carry bag.

"Are you Jane?"

All pleasantries were exchanged but both of us knew I did not want to be there. Who would? This time last week my life was just dandy thank you very much. Fast forward one week and there I was standing in the reception of a small hospital with a wad of scans under my arm, getting the pity look from everyone there who were silently saying to themselves, "I'm glad it's not me."

As I got ready for surgery, the breast care nurse presented me with what looked like a novel of brochures and leaflets on breast cancer. I politely declined the bulging bag of information, saying I would be fine and I didn't need to read anything because, firstly, it was going to scare the shit of me, and secondly, I quite liked the fact I knew nothing. That way I could at least try and process in my mind how the hell I had gotten there.

I likened it to when I had children. I read nothing about giving birth, I didn't go to classes, I barely spoke to anyone about it. I didn't want to hear anyone's horror stories and totally believed *it will be what it will be*. I may have been naïve or stubborn—both probably—but I certainly didn't need a whole lot of literature about breast cancer to haul home with me. That bag sat there untouched. When I left the hospital, the pink bag stayed exactly where it had been placed. Good riddance.

I couldn't wait to get home to have a decent cup of tea and a cigarette.

I realise now, in the wonderful state of hindsight, that I was in denial. The meaning of denial is, "In which a person is faced with a fact that is too uncomfortable to accept and rejects it instead, insisting that it is not true despite what may be overwhelming evidence."

Over the next week, I carried on with life like I always had, did household chores, ran errands, and caught up with friends; in my mind nothing had happened.

I recovered remarkably well from surgery, surprising even myself. It was OK, I was OK; I could get on with my life. Medical people were starting to call me; I didn't answer any of their phone calls. Appointments were being made for me and I didn't want to go. I just carried on like nothing had happened.

Good, I thought. *I have my life back.*

# CHAPTER 3

I finally went to my surgeon's follow up appointment, really only because my husband came with me. That was the last time anyone accompanied me to any appointment—the only way I was going to get through this was on my own. I loathed having anyone with me. I still feel this way. I am fiercely independent and my own warrior. I do not need anyone to make decisions for me; I am quite capable, thank you very much.

I was determined to do it my way, and on my own terms. It was not a new way of thinking for me; I am neither an introvert, nor someone who doesn't want the help and support of people, but this was my problem and I truly didn't want to burden anyone with something that was mine to own.

It was *my* cancer.

No one could *tell* me anything about dealing with cancer. Nobody I knew had cancer; none of my family, none of my friends. There was nothing out there about how to think about, or deal with it.

How did a normal person do it?

I bought Jennifer Saunders' book, *Bonkers*, because I knew she had had breast cancer, and although she dedicates only a few chapters in her book to it, she wrote in a way I could totally relate to. I could identify with her for some reason, although she lives in a different country, and she is a famous comedian, but her experiences resonated with me. I read those chapters five times. I wanted to take a leaf out of her book.

I particularly loved her take on drinking and chemo, if your body was going to be injected with poison you might as well have a glass of wine, you have so much crap in your body anyway. Now that was a take on cancer I liked, and actually, I was starting to think it might be OK.

I had a referral to see a specialist, time was ticking away, and I couldn't put off the fact I was going to need treatment—a lot of it—but, I had a holiday to organise; I was leaving in three weeks time—shit!

I had organised my dad's 70th birthday to be celebrated in Bali. I had sixteen members of my family descending on the island in less than three weeks' time. I had planned a birthday dinner at the villas where we were staying, and I was going, come hell or high water.

If I dropped out, the game was up. I would have to tell people I had cancer and I wasn't ready for that, not at all. I have heard a few times, people have had cruises booked, or once in a lifetime holidays planned, only to be knocked down by a cancer diagnosis. What awful timing. I wasn't going to cancel, I was taking my holiday just how I planned it and nothing was going to stop me.

People do cancel holidays, and I wonder why? What possibly can't be delayed for one or two weeks? I think it is imperative before facing cancer treatment to have something to look forward to and enjoy. I obviously had that cancer growing for a period of time and I was still around, what was another two weeks going to matter? I had had surgery; it was technically gone, why the rush?

I struggled with the concept. Why do the medical professionals rush you so much? Why is everything at lightning and break neck speed? It is way too much to take in all at once. My head was a whirlwind of information and I understood practically none of it. I had landed on a planet that was so foreign to me it couldn't possibly be true; who were all these people telling me what to do?

My head was in a spin, leaving me so overwhelmed, I wanted to stop the world and get off.

Boarding that plane was like entering Alice in Wonderland. Down the rabbit hole into the life I knew well, the life I wanted back. I was me again, stepping out of the airport and taking in a lungful of that beautiful, humid air, filled with frangipanis and warmth.

Ahh…that was more like it. The paradise was where I belonged right then, not at hospitals and seeing specialists with their nasty news and their telling me what to do. I was in control. I was with my beautiful family, my husband and my children. There was no place on earth I would rather be than in that tropical paradise.

I was happier than I had been in weeks, thank God. The past three weeks were just a dream—a horrible one—and in Bali I didn't have to face what was happening. I was in blissful denial, I didn't care, either.

None of my extended family knew about my cancer, and I wasn't going to say a word. That would give the cancer some sort of right to be in my life, I was not going to be identified by it – it was not me. I didn't want anyone to think any different of me, and I certainly didn't want anyone feeling sorry for me. Not only that, if I told anyone I would be hijacking my dad's birthday celebrations. I was quite clear in my mind; cancer would not define me or my life. I was pretending, I know that now, but I soldiered on and put a smile on my face.

I couldn't wait to see everyone. Family members started arriving at different times throughout the next two days and we had started a social media group to keep in contact with each other. We had booked a fantastic villa, with separate bedrooms and a full sized pool in the middle. The garden was filled with tropical plants and flowers and the frangipani trees were hanging over the pool and dropping their beautifully scented flowers into the water. It was magical. That was our home for the next two weeks.

The afternoon was sultry and a storm was brewing in the distance; the weather hot and humid. As we took shelter under our pergola, I could see fish calmly swimming around the small moat we had between our outdoor kitchen and bedroom villas. It was mesmerising. I would catch myself daydreaming, then the thoughts of the last three weeks would come back into the forefront of my mind.

It never once occurred to me I should tell my family. I had to shield them from the awfulness that was my life. They didn't need to know what was going on.

I had to be careful with what I wore, I still had a rather large skin bandage covering the top of my left breast and I had to wear less than fetching crop tops that had no support under everything.

That had been a problem after surgery; there was nothing affordable out there to accommodate women who had breast surgery. I ended up buying a rather hideous pack of three crop tops from a discount department store that did the job for all day comfort, but had no support, and the thick, wide straps made it impossible to cover up with anything other than a kaftan. I had to wear those crop tops 24/7; as soon as I took them off the surgery scar would start twinging from not being locked in the constraints of the stretchy material.

My lumpectomy scar was quite high up, as it turned out. When I first felt the flat ropey lump in my breast it felt like it was attached to the top of my rib cage, right up in the top left quarter. As it turned out, it was fortuitous as there has been very little change to the shape of my breast after having surgery; the left one sat only slightly higher than the right, and really who could tell in a bra—or crop top—for that matter?

Most women don't have exactly the same sized breasts anyway, so I didn't feel they looked vastly different. That was a relief and something I was very happy about, even though my tumour was 3.5cm (which is considered to be on the large side) it had been scooped out perfectly, and I only had a thin pink line where the stitches had dissolved underneath. The scar was neat and ran across the top of my breast like an upside down smiling face.

I had to be careful, no swimming unless it was in the safety of our villa because I couldn't hide it. It was poking up out of my bikini like a beacon, one glance at that and it was all over, too many questions. I purposely went and bought a few new dresses that covered the evidence of surgery.

I can't say I didn't struggle with the charade. It was exhausting being on alert to anything that may have given me away. I was obviously still recovering; I arrived in Bali exactly three weeks after and I was tired from the surgery, the anaesthetic, and the heavy mental state of being diagnosed with cancer. I didn't want that to show, I had to be involved in all the activities, lunches, dinners, I couldn't be seen not joining in. It was imperative to being the organiser. The birthday kept me busy, which I relished; it took my mind off everything else. I was happy in that space—I couldn't think about the alternative—but it was exhausting.

Back home, and the stark reality of it all really hit me. I wanted to go back to Bali where I didn't have to think about cancer, I wanted sunshine and roses and puppies! Anything but cancer.

Not for the first time, I wanted my old life back; I didn't want to go anywhere near the hospitals, doctors, specialists—none of them. Bali was such a haven, a moment in time that I could be me, and rest, relax, enjoy my life. I wanted to be back in my happy place in Bali.

I finally made an appointment with a specialist and dragged my sorry arse to his medical rooms. I so did not want to be there. As he ushered me in, he was looking behind me.

"Is someone with you?"

I cut him off straight away, "I don't need anyone."

I had been sitting there for less than a few minutes when I became totality fixated on the fact that he had holes in his clothes. One in the pocket of his suit jacket, and one on the elbow where the fabric had worn away from over wear.

How does someone who charges $480 an hour have holes in his clothes?

I work in men's fashion, I know that suits don't cost that much. Two appointments and he could afford a new one.

I couldn't focus on anything he was saying. I was mesmerised by the holes, and couldn't help wonder why he would choose to put that particular suit on in the morning and think no one would notice. How bizarre. I'm no clothes snob but I was there as a potential patient and all I could think of was that he was not equipped to look after me.

Like the last specialist, he took to scribbling on bits of paper with lines, charts, percentages, tick boxes, all of which made no sense to me. What was it with the paper drawings? It wasn't kindergarten, it was my life being reduced to a few squiggles on a scrap piece of paper.

It's funny what you do remember. Apart from the holes in his clothes, he said, "Well at least you aren't on your own, I have a patient who has no one."

How exactly was that reassuring? What was that about? That

I have a husband and children; what did that have to do with anything? Who were these people? No matter what, this was about me and I expected to be treated as a person, not compared to someone else. I deserved definite clarity and well-informed empathy from all specialists.

He was not robust, in my view. I was seeking the best for me, and he wasn't that. It was crap, and I was feeling crappier by the hour. If he was supposed to make me feel better and get a plan underway, then it failed. I felt lost.

I spent the rest of that appointment clutching my handbag and staring out the window. The days were getting cooler as the autumn weather had started turning the leaves to a golden hue. I remember the view from the office, up several storeys overlooking the city. A perfect view for any other time, but who wanted to look at it when being told you need chemotherapy from a man in a worn suit?

I could sense he was getting agitated. I was not behaving like a perfect patient, but who does? And who says you have to? I sensed that he thought I should be the one complying; I was having none of it, he could stuff his treatment up his worn out jumper!

After nearly two hours, I left, stood on the street and lit a cigarette. I wasn't going back there.

Next!

# CHAPTER 4

I needed another referral. Shit.

In the meantime, I had been sent for a myriad of tests. There was not one bit of any of those tests that was not anxiety ridden or completely terrifying. CT scans, bone scans, ultrasounds, heart tests...the list went on, and so did the money coming out of my account.

I had yet to meet anyone in the process who gave a flying shit (there was one, but more on her later). I was just another number.

No one cared that I had a full on claustrophobic anxiety attack with foreboding machines practically touching my face while the staff warned me if I didn't settle down they would have to inject me with Valium.

What the? Did I hear that correctly? Where was I, in some sort of horror film?

I wasn't just anxious, I was sweating, my heart was jumping out of my chest and at any minute I was terrified I would pass out or shit my pants. Neither scenario was inviting to say the least, and for the first time in my life, I was totally out of my head, literally.

Oh. My. God!

It took me the rest of the day, and ten cigarettes accompanied by a strong coffee, to settle down. Neither of those are what I would recommend but it worked for me that day. I wasn't shaking from anxiety, but from nicotine and caffeine. I was six weeks post-surgery with no plan. I was starting to shit myself. I needed to do something.

I decided to read the Cancer Council website information on breast cancer; I downloaded all 120 pages of it.

Jeez, why could they not just write that stuff in a nut shell?

It's so much commitment to read all that information when you are in denial anyway. Usually an avid reader, it sent me into a spin. I didn't want to learn as much as I could because it scared me. It was all medical stuff that, one, I didn't understand, two, half of it didn't apply to me, and three, was downright depressing.

It was information overload; I didn't want a bar of it. I know some people want as much information as they can get their hands on, that wasn't me at all. I couldn't face it, what I didn't know couldn't hurt me. I could deal with the information in small bites, if the specialists told me something that I thought was applicable to me then I would take that in, but not all the general stuff out there.

In fact, nothing applies to you. You are on your own, and no one can know what will happen to you, only you. It was a very lonely time, and reading about everyone else's side effects, complications, types of cancer, only sent me into the abyss. The black hole of fear.

I again dragged my sorry arse to the next specialist. My appointment was at 3.15pm, and at 4.30pm when I was still in the waiting room with no one, including the reception staff, bothering to tell me anything, I up and left. End of story. Again, how could this person be in charge of my treatment when they clearly don't own a watch?

I suppose this is endemic in a health world of unpredictable events, but it's horrible when you have cancer—awful in itself.

Do those people care? What if I was their wife? Their sister? Their mum? Would they treat them with the same disdain or lack of compassion? Or lack of a watch?

OK. I was starting to sense something: was it me? I was weeks past my surgery now, and still no plan. I didn't know how to behave in that scenario. It was so out of my comfort zone, I was fed up with it already and I still had a year of treatment to contemplate. I couldn't do it. I couldn't even find a specialist.

I was starting to think since I felt fine, I was not sick. I don't need all this stuff. Sounds like overkill to me. I finally got through the wads of paper from the Cancer Council, the course of treatments, side effects, long terms effects, and it was like a horror movie. I deleted the PDF from my phone.

# CHAPTER 5

I finally found a specialist I liked. Well, not like in the way you like your hairdresser, but she was ten times better than anyone else I had seen. She was a tick boxer, which I didn't mind because at least she was organised. And she definitely owned a watch, she was never late.

It probably seems strange to anyone else, but the time thing really bothered me. No one's time is more important than anyone else's, I don't care what anyone says. It is disrespectful when people make you wait, it's like they see themselves as more important. I don't like that. I certainly don't like it when you are talking about cancer patients.

I just wanted someone to be kind and empathetic. If I were a specialist, and I chose a profession to heal and treat cancer patients, I would at least be nice to my patients. My girlfriends told me there is no accounting for human failings sometimes. I was under the illusion that everyone would be super sympathetic, but no, unfortunately, that hadn't been my experience. The specialists I saw seemed to just go through the motions, just like a script. You gain a sense of feeling like you are not important enough, not a serious enough case.

"For God's sake, I have cancer!" I wanted to shout at them all.

So I got myself a specialist, what then?

"Ready for chemo?" she asked as I walked through the door to her rooms.

She had to be joking; who would ever think they were ready for chemo?

Even the word scared me, it was worse than the word cancer. I knew no one, and I mean no one who had ever had chemo, and all I remember at that time is how sick people became from it. That if the cancer didn't kill you, there was a possibility the chemotherapy could. How on earth did I get there?

There was no time in my life I ever thought I would have to face the realisation that I needed chemotherapy. Who does?

There I was, facing over a year of treatment, with no idea how it would make me feel. It is so unknowable, so daunting. I wanted to run out of that room as fast as I could and never go back. The fear of the unknown is terrifying; I had no one to talk to who had been down the same road.

The specialists all talk in a hurried, almost-whisper about treatment. I could not work out if they were trying to be concerned, or trying to scare the shit out of me. Their matter of fact manner was disturbing. I wished they would just come out and say, "This is crap and there is nothing I can say that will make you feel better." Actually, telling me straight would have made me feel better. It would have been at least more human.

It was two of my girlfriend's birthdays as there is only eleven days between them. They had organised a dinner out on a Sunday night at the local burger bar. I still hadn't told anyone about my cancer. No one. It had been weeks now since I was diagnosed. On my way to meeting my friends, I also had no intention of telling them. Business as usual, a few laughs, plenty of wine and food and generally a great catch up on everyone's gossip. I didn't want it to be any different.

As I sat there with my four dearest friends, I burst into tears. I couldn't do it, I couldn't not tell them, I have known these beautiful people for ten years. I ended up blurting it out, "I have breast cancer."

We held hands across the table like otters and we all cried. The other customers at the burger bar were starting to stare and the staff were wondering what on earth a group of forty-something's were blubbering at.

But I finally felt like I had a weight off my shoulders. I clearly needed to tell someone. Not just anyone; people who would truly understand and be there for me, not for themselves with their own health agendas.

I had deliberately not told members of my family. My family has a history of overreacting to health crises, I didn't want to be the centre of attention, and I didn't want to have to explain anything. I just wanted to be able to talk about how I felt, and understand that I was still me and would be absolutely fine.

Never during that time did I think I was going to pop my clogs, not once. I knew that for sure. I just didn't know how I was going to get through the next fifteen months of treatment. That was a mountain I had to climb and my back was against the wall, the only way was forward, but I didn't want to take the steps. I was almost frozen in the fear of all that impending treatment. It sounded terrifying, who in their right mind would want to do it? Are you joking?

Chemo was to start on Friday, and I was totally terrified. I ate nothing for the three days prior, only coffee and cigarettes—again not conductive to cancer treatment. Thursday night and I was sick to my stomach, I couldn't sleep. My appointment was at 10.30am, and it was the slowest countdown ever. Worse than a child waiting for Santa Claus.

My girlfriends had done a 'chemo roster' and I cried when they told me. They said there was no way I was going to do chemo alone—not a chance—even though it was what I wanted. I realise now that was the best gift ever; having them with me, week in and week out, was the only thing about treatment that I looked forward to. Hours spent with my girlfriends.

I remember at the time being desperate to find my inner peace, desperate for my mind to calm itself. I started to scour my bookshelves for anything I could to make some sense of my fear.

I dragged out an old copy of a book I had read and used when I was suffering a rather bad case of anxiety a few years before. *Letting it Go* by Bev Aisbett (not the Disney *Let it go* version).

They are a series of books written and illustrated by Bev, and really are marvellous. The cartoon drawings make it feel just a little bit humorous with a serious message. Bev Aisbett is a survivor of panic disorder and in the books shares how she overcame "IT" (her name for your panic) and what strategies she used to change her mindset. She talks about how we blame ourselves, others or divine judgement when bad things happen to us.

I was definitely blaming myself. My thoughts were like a runaway train, speeding ahead and looking like they would hurl off the bridge into the river below. I was replaying everything over and over in my mind like a broken record; my thoughts of the future were being clouded by my experiences of the past. All I could think about were the 'bad' things. I couldn't think of the good, the fact that I had early breast cancer should have been a blessing, but I wasn't thinking that way. I was so doom and gloom. All I could think about was that I had cancer. Me. *I* had it. How come I had to have it?

My out of control thoughts were affecting me in every way—not only my mind, but my body. I was exhausted just from my thoughts playing a crazy song over and over again in my head.

Bev writes about a 'source' in her book, and I very much like this concept, we all have a source, it's our original perfection. She talks about how throughout our lives we keep hitting blocks to our source, whether that be pain or trauma and for some of us, that means hitting those blocks time and time again, because as humans we are slow learners.

Indeed we are, I am certainly a slow learner in this department. I tried to remember back over the few months before I was diagnosed. I was in a pretty shitty space really, now that I had time to reflect upon it.

Life the year before my diagnosis was coasting along, it was Christmas time, I wasn't unhappy—far from it—but I know I just didn't feel right in myself. I was doing all of my usual things leading up to Christmas; catching up with friends, family, and winding down at work for a two week break. All usual stuff.

My life was as hectic as the next person's, and around Christmas it ramped up, so that meant more late nights out, more glasses of champagne, more social smoking, more of everything.

We were travelling for Christmas so there seemed an urgency to see everyone before we left. When we finally reached our Christmas destination, I was relieved to be able to slow down. But I still didn't feel right.

I had dizzy spells that made me feel quite nauseous. My head felt like it was floating in clouds; a weird sensation that I couldn't put my finger on, like when you have morphine after an operation, you know you are awake but your senses have failed you and everything is dreamy. It really is quite an unnerving feeling. I would feel like that at least three to four times a day, sometimes for an hour at a time. I knew it couldn't be normal. Maybe it was what a 'block' feels like. Now I think back to that time, I had more than a block. Bev says that everything happens for a reason and that pain is a motivator – I had of course heard this before but I was really starting to believe that something just wasn't quite right.

When we returned from Christmas, I knew I had to find out what was happening to me. My 'source' had gone AWOL. I realise now I was stressed, my anxiety had started to rear its ugly head again, and I was feeling 'sick' even though I had no physical symptoms that could be measured. How do you tell someone in the medical profession that you have a blockage in your 'source'?

I went for dozens of tests, all confirming there was nothing wrong with me. Heart tests, blood tests, etc. none of them came back with anything conclusive. I was starting to think I was becoming a hypochondriac. I went to see them four times in a week. I don't think I had even been to the doctors four times in the last year and there I was practically living on their doorstep.

It is said that stress begins with negative thoughts; I think I had my fair share of them. I got testy if someone pushed in front of me at the supermarket and would give them a deathly stare. I sometimes spoke poorly about a relative or friend. Other times I would beat myself up over spending too much money on frivolous things; I was sucking the positive things out of my life and replacing them with negative ones.

I never thought I would have climbed over that fence, but I was jumpy all of the time. I would do crazy things, like get up in the middle of the night because I heard a sound and rush about the house checking doors, peering out of windows, and making sure my children were still in bed. I was becoming scared – scared of life, scared of myself, I was high on stress all the time. I recognise now, that it was the start of the 'worst and best day of my life'.

# CHAPTER 6

Chemo day, my girlfriends were so gorgeous. They said I could sleep, read, or have my arse whipped at connect four or scrabble; all sounded so much better than being injected with chemotherapy. Contemplating my immune system firing on all cylinders, and the chemo going in to thwart my cancer beast, was the only thing that kept me going. I had to trust the wonders of the modern medical world, the miraculous power of the human body to repair itself, and the power of friendship with their will to help me through.

None of us had ever faced such a health crises, we were all inexperienced and bewildered by the medical system, and how on earth I got cancer.

That was the worst drive ever, the first day of chemo. I wanted to run, and run a long way from there, a long way from my strange new life.

On my first treatment, the staff gave me a wad of information on side effects. I am not kidding it was twenty-five pages long! Twenty-five pages of side effects!

I remember thinking to myself, *why on earth would you read that*? I was going to scare myself senseless. I threw it all in the bin; I couldn't bring myself to go through it. I know I was ignorant, I didn't care, and ignorance was bliss as far as I saw it.

Oh, God!

Nothing can prepare you for walking into an oncology ward for your first day of chemotherapy, that is one place I never want to be again, EVER. The only positive part was that the day oncology at my local hospital is really a very lovely space, and the staff were all angels.

It is all white with large windows overlooking the park. A very calm space where, if you don't think about the fact you're in an oncology ward, you would be happy to sit and read in the beautiful light. The April weather was cool but the sun was shining through the enormous windows and even though people were milling around and assisting patients, there was a sense of calm, a sense that I would be alright with these people.

I was certainly not used to being anywhere like it. I had never been in an oncology ward; there were countless machines, all beeping a chorus of warning sounds, but it still had an air of efficiency about it.

Oncology nurses are angels—no two ways about it. I have never felt more at ease in a hospital, (and I have had some truly horrendous experiences, resulting in a most likely irrational fear, developed over many years).

I welcomed those beautiful people into my world, I could sense their compassion and they totally 'got' how I was feeling. Finally, people in the medical profession who cared enough for it to radiate from their souls. Not once did I ever feel like a number, a distraction, a burden, a source of angst; they were there to help me and as far as I was concerned I was the only person in the ward. That was how well they took care of me. Nothing was a bother, nothing was too much trouble. Thank God. I needed those people to get me through the next fifteen months of treatment. And they did.

Luckily, I am not afraid of needles. I am ever so thankful for that because it was at the start of a very long period of people sticking me with them.

I had been warned about chemo and veins, but when the nurses tell you your veins may 'pop', 'roll', or 'disappear altogether', it sends you into a stratosphere of anxiety.

So, I was faced with the very real problem of not having any viable veins in my right arm, even after a few treatments of chemo—what the?

The nurses told me they would keep using the cannula until my veins gave up. I mean, how long would that take?

They couldn't tell me. My veins could take a permanent holiday in a few weeks' time, or never. It made me a bit cranky, all the, "Well it may happen, or it may not happen", and, "We don't know if this will work for you."

There was not a thing in the world I would keep doing if it didn't work. Would I keep banging my head against a brick wall if it wasn't doing anything? Of course not! But you are expected to sign up for months and months of treatment that may or may not work, and by the way, will probably make you sicker.

Who signs up for that?

Well I did, and there I was sitting in a place I never thought I would ever be, being injected with poison and being told my veins probably won't be up to the challenge. Chemo was getting worse by the minute.

In hindsight (which is a wonderful thing), I would have had a port put in. The option was not discussed with me at all, I found out about them from another patient in the day oncology, but by that time I was half way through my treatment and I really didn't want to have surgery or a general anaesthetic again. So I decided not to. My veins survived, but I wished someone had told me about it much earlier on, like when I had my lumpectomy; it would have at least helped me with all those inconvenient trips to the toilet during treatment.

I did, however, sign up for the scalp cooling, because there was not a chance I was going to lose my hair. That was a definite. How could I keep my diagnosis to myself when all my hair had fallen out? I wasn't ready for that, and I was terrified of losing my hair. It seems vain, it seems trivial, but it is something I couldn't get past. If I could not save my hair, I wasn't having chemotherapy. I was not changing my mind. If I started and the scalp cooling wasn't working, I would stop chemotherapy treatment. That was a given. I was determined to stick out the scalp cooling, I didn't care if it was going to add three hours to my treatment (what else would I be doing?), and I was prepared for the brain freeze.

Before any treatments started I was hooked up to the scalp cooling machine which is quite the pa lava. First, your hair has to be wet and coated in conditioner before they put a very snug fitting cap on your head, which is not just tight, it is a vice. It cannot be loose otherwise it won't work. Those chilled channels in the cap need to be right on your scalp. My girlfriend told me that I belonged in the water polo team. It was exactly what I looked like; I could compete at the Olympics, it was very sporty and green.

Then, you have another Velcro cap put over the top that adds even more vice-like treatment. At that stage my face was contorted from the tight straps around my chin, and I looked like I had been stung by a bee (whilst playing water polo).

Next, you are connected by two tubes to the freezer. That was by far the weirdest feeling. All of a sudden I felt the channels filling up and it was starting to get very cold. In fact, those machines 'chill' your scalp to about ten degrees; which might seem OK if you were outside in ten degrees, with your winter woollies on, but not so much when it is restricted to your scalp.

For that reason, the nurses gave me a heated blanket which was by far the best thing ever. It was made of paper and hot air was channelled in through a little pump. I wanted one to take home.

I was hooked up to the scalp cooling, submerged in my cocoon, and generally feeling very sleepy when they started the infusions. And wow there was a lot of them.

Three lots of pre-medication, one chemotherapy, and one biological therapy (Herceptin). I was going to be there for a while. The mixture of a freezing head and a cocktail of drugs was starting to take its toll. I was sleepy and trying desperately to keep my eyes open to talk to my girlfriend who was so generously giving me her time. It was a long day to sit in the oncology ward just watching someone sleep.

Another wonderful service at the chemo ward is the roving beautician. It was an amazing service. I had never heard of beauticians in hospitals—I learnt a lot that day.

What angels they are. You can choose from a manicure, pedicure, or massage. Wow. All part of my stay in the day oncology ward. Well, I thought. *I am going to take full advantage of this*! I had my fingernails painted every week thereafter. Which was probably just as well, because after seven weeks of chemo my nails started going a rather strange brown colour.

My first treatment passed with no real issues and the seven hours went remarkably fast, mainly because I had passed out wrapped up in a hot bubble with ice on top.

## CHAPTER 7

No one tells you that the steroids they give you make you wired. Not just a little bit, a lot! I couldn't sleep at all that night. I had gone from comatose to the Energizer bunny, with eyes like saucers, compelled to start cleaning the kitchen. What was in that stuff? I had never taken any form of steroid before and I couldn't believe I wasn't tired at all. I lay awake all night, my mind going around in circles leaving me with way too much time to over-think everything. Not a great combination, really. I was trying to stop the flood of irrational and fearful thoughts and instead they gave me something that made my brain switch on for days on end. I didn't even have that luxury of going to sleep and forgetting about the situation I was in. It was a recurring nightmare all day long.

I was feeling very sorry for myself. I still really wanted to fly solo. My girlfriends were my team and I could manage the small circle of four friends, my husband, and children. Anymore and it was too public. I wasn't ready for the questions, the sympathy, or the pity.

My girlfriend sent me a message that day, "Sympathy? You know where you find sympathy? It's in the dictionary between sod off and syphilis". What a dose of reality!

I did not need to do anything faster than I wanted to. It was at my pace, my time frame, my comfort zone. I chose how to do it.

Three days after my first treatment, I actually felt OK. No nausea, which was the biggest worry I had, I hated feeling like I wanted to throw up. My girlfriend was totally convinced that chemo caused nausea during treatment; in the actual moment she was planning to hold a bucket and my hair.

I felt blessed, what a relief. I could have a glass of wine. My menu: water, wine, water, wine, water, wine... isn't that how you become the messiah? Turning water into wine? The simple life luxury of having a glass of wine was very welcome. No one wants to spend time in a chemo chair, and that glass of wine made my day.

I had been getting a lot of health tips, all in good faith but, nonetheless, irritating when I knew I was healthy anyway. But I took to juicing beetroot, celery, and ginger, as I had read that they were cancer fighting foods. Who even knows? But they tasted good and I was feeling physically well, so I stuck with it.

It is an interesting conundrum, lifestyle risks. Why can no one answer the question of who gets cancer? There is so much out there that makes sense, and makes no sense. It's nonsense!

Nobody fits the criteria according to the experts—I know I certainly didn't. I wasn't overweight, I'm not diabetic, and always exercising. I eat well, I have had children, blah, blah, blah, and the list goes on.

Most women who have been diagnosed with breast cancer are healthy; we live our lives in moderation with a balanced diet and a glass of wine here and there. It's just common sense. There is no rhyme or reason; dumb bad luck doesn't discriminate.

Any woman, from any walk of life, can get cancer. I would really love it if the experts stopped publishing lists of risk factors because they don't make any sense. When you are awake at 3am in the morning, tossing and turning in your bed, and your mind is racing ahead at a million miles an hour you do not want to think, *if only I had breastfed my baby I wouldn't have breast cancer.*

Ridiculous I know, but the so-called risk factors only make us feel worse. It's the 'what ifs' and 'what if I hads' all over again. It is so stressful to keep the loop of thoughts going around in your head. According to the experts and their lists I should not have got breast cancer at all, but I did. How was that explained? I had no known genetic cause.

I guess I will never know, nothing will change that fact and I need to learn to live with it. But it would be helpful if we weren't constantly bombarded by data that doesn't help you accept what has happened.

I received a chemotherapy show bag from my girlfriends—or should I say, chemotherapy contraband kit. Each item could be used when there was a relevant situation.

There were three pairs of plastic glamour glasses, sweets, hand sanitiser, creams and lotions, worry dolls, and stress balls. All great things to relieve anxiety and turn an awful situation into something I could look forward to.

I wore those crazy glasses to make the cold cap not look quite so ridiculous. I couldn't believe once a week I would dress up in novelty plastic glasses and a water polo cap to take photos of myself in the chemo chair. You don't ever think about trying to cheer yourself up by wearing plastic glasses with ridiculous guitars on the rims. I know one day I will look back and laugh, just not right now.

My second week of chemo was on my daughter's birthday. She was turning twelve. I had given birth to her exactly twelve years ago in the same hospital that I was sitting in receiving treatment. It was not lost on me. I cried. I cried because twelve years ago it was the best day of my life to welcome my new baby girl, while twelve years later I was sitting in an oncology ward hooked up to frightful machines and dealing with a breast cancer diagnosis.

I wanted to be with my beautiful girl, I wanted to celebrate with her on her special day, not be there. I never wanted my children to see me in the oncology ward so they never came with me. I couldn't do it. I protected them from seeing me in that place. It would have been too confronting for them, and for me, too close to home.

I struggled on the days my husband accompanied me. I didn't want him to come either. I knew he wanted to be there for me, but he couldn't do anything. He was helpless to even comfort me through any of that awfulness. I didn't want him to see me like that; I felt like I had let him down. I was flawed, I was sick, I was not the same anymore. I had cancer.

He would ask me every day how I was feeling and while it was very lovely of him to keep asking after me, I got tired of answering the same thing and I became irritated. I just wanted to be left alone. I didn't want to keep answering the silly questions; I was fine!

Really though, I didn't want to be bothered by small talk about whether I felt sick, because of course I felt like crap. I had constant diarrhoea, bloody noses, fatigue, and I was being systematically poisoned every week. What do you reckon I felt like?

I didn't want to feel that way towards him. He loves me, and I know he wanted to help, but I had to do it myself.

My days were consumed with constant thoughts about cancer; I just couldn't get them out of my head. It was all consuming, never ending, circling around in my mind; I felt mentally sick and overwhelmed everyday even though I was distracting myself at work. My thoughts would drift off all the time, how did this become my life? I was happy before, I didn't want to do it. I didn't want to go to the hospital, I didn't want to have chemo, I didn't want to see specialists, I didn't want anything to do with it.

Stop, stop, stop!

After the second week of chemo my hair starting falling out. Not the hair on my head but everywhere else. It was not unexpected, but in the same token quite unnerving when I had spent most of my life trying to get rid of body hair. And there it was, just falling out. Wow. If there was a way to harness it without getting cancer I would have totally been on board with that as a hair removal technique. The hair under my arms was the first to go. *Handy*, I thought. *I can wear singlet tops now and not have to worry about underarm hair*! Except it was autumn and I wasn't about to be wearing sleeveless tops. Bummer.

By far the weirdest and strangest occurrence in the body hair department was losing my pubic hair. I had never been a fan of the Brazilian—ouch, no thanks! But almost one by one the hair just fell out. I saw it in the shower recess travelling towards the plug hole. It came out in clumps, so for a time there, it looked like I had attacked it with a pair of rose pruners. By the fourth week, it was all but completely gone; I found the remainder of it piled up inside my underpants. I hadn't seen myself like that since primary school.

I didn't know what to think looking at myself in the bathroom mirror. I had all of my head hair, but not a single hair in any other place on my body, to go with a pair of boobs that were slightly lopsided. I never would have thought that would be the reflection staring back at me, and I didn't know whether to laugh or cry. I did however, do a happy dance for not having to shave my legs for the foreseeable future.

My girlfriends continued to support me and my 'chemo roster', week in week out. The time went both quickly and slowly. I just wanted the nightmare to be over already. Why did I have to sit in that oncology chair? It just wasn't fair.

My girlfriend had recently returned from a holiday in New York and she was eager to show me her photos when we were holed up in the hospital for six hours. I wanted to be excited to see them, I had never been to New York, but I found it so hard to be enthusiastic. She was showing me them on her phone as I sat with my head in a freezing cap with tubes running poison through my veins. I couldn't think of things like holidays. I was insanely jealous. I wanted to go to New York, I wanted to be as far away from this place as I could.

I hated the fact every Friday I had to front up at the oncology ward; it was so hard to keep a smile on my face. Inside I was hurting, I cried in my sleep, I cried for a life I had lost and I cried because I didn't know if I could beat this. What would I do if all this treatment didn't work? I was a wreck.

# CHAPTER 8

I felt strangely compelled to talk to my neighbour. I knew her, but not well. We waved to each other in the street but otherwise it was over the fence banter like Tim 'the tool man' Taylor. I had told very few people about my diagnosis, even at that time I found it hard to tell people. What do you say?

Nice morning. Oh, by the way, I have cancer. See you later.

I couldn't do it. I was still burying my head in the sand. I just kept my rather big secret to myself. I wanted to live a normal life. Fiercely independent, it wasn't me to shout it from the rooftops. But I knew my neighbour had her own experience with cancer.

Her mum, only three years ago, had been diagnosed with stage three breast cancer, and undergone a mastectomy, chemo, and radiation. My neighbour had supported her through the whole treatment so I knew she would be a good person to talk to as someone who had navigated that path with a loved one.

I knocked on her door and her husband answered and ushered me into their family room. She was on the phone but waved at me to sit down. When she had finished her phone call she said, "Nice to see you Jane." But I could sense she was thinking, *why are you here? You haven't knocked on my door for years.*

She organised a glass of wine and we sat in her front room.

I just blurted it out.

"I have breast cancer and I had chemotherapy yesterday and I have to have it every week."

OK, there is was. Out in the open to my neighbour. Not my family, or close friends; my neighbour who I barely knew and was not in my inner circle.

I am so glad I told her. She was so supportive and said, "One day at a time."

I didn't know just how apt that would be until much later. At that time, I was taking every hour as it came, but she was right. Little steps, and tomorrow was a new day. We talked for two hours about everything and anything. I felt relieved to have spoken to someone in length about how I was feeling and she knew the right words to say to me. Her mum had come through treatment with flying colours and she was living a full and happy life on the coast in Queensland.

If her mum could do it, so could I.

The very next day my neighbour left a lovely plant outside my front door at the exact time my parents arrived to visit. My mum asked why my neighbour was leaving such a lovely and generous gift and I said it was because I had helped her out with something, and she was grateful for the help. Another white lie to my family.

That same neighbour recommended yoga to me a few weeks after my diagnosis. I had never done yoga, ever. I wasn't really that interested, but she gave me a name of a local yoga studio. She said she likened negative thoughts to a snow globe; your head can be like someone is shaking that snow globe all the time and white fuzzy stuff is flying around constantly. By practising yoga, the white fuzzy stuff stays at the bottom.

Yoga was the furthest thing from my mind right then, but considering my mind was rampant with the most unhelpful and fearful thoughts, I thought maybe it would help.

I had to do something. I had become another person. I was angry, I was sad, and worse, I had become suicidal. For all intents and purposes I was living inside my head, a life only just holding together.

I was terrified every Thursday night before the Fridays I had chemo treatment, and I used to stand in the shower on Friday mornings before my girlfriend picked me up, crying uncontrollably about why my life had become so awful. I used to sit in the bottom of the shower praying that someone would just shoot me, then I wouldn't have to face this, it would all go away.

I hated my life, I hated the fact I had cancer, I couldn't face the next twelve months of treatment, it was too much to bear. I know I didn't ask for help, I wanted so bad to sort it out myself because I knew somewhere deep down inside I knew I had 'it' in me, I had done it before. That warrior woman was somewhere, I just had to find her.

For people who don't suffer from anxiety or a cancer diagnosis, there is nothing they could say to make you feel any better. It was a viscous cycle of dreadful thoughts and the fear of dying. I really knew nothing about cancer, all I knew was, I had it and it could kill me. No one in the medical profession could tell me my survival chances. If a specialist couldn't tell you with all their years of training and knowledge how could anyone? I felt so lost, so out of control.

I would finish my shower, load my eyes up on drops so no one could see I had been crying, patch up my skin with tinted moisturiser, and emerge from the bathroom with no one having a clue I'd had a complete meltdown.

# CHAPTER 9

Who would have thought something that has been around for thousands of years could be the answer for me?

I called the studio and booked in for the free sessions. When I turned up to the studio, it was the owner's home in a downstairs conversion looking out into the garden. It was autumn, and straight away I could feel the calmness of the space.

I knew nothing about yoga, not a thing. All I could remember was my mum had a friend in the 70's that was some sort of yogi, and she was very much the alternative, broad-bean-eating type who had Llamas in her back garden.

But the studio was lovely. No broad beans or incense in sight! It was really rather modern, and as I set myself up on my mat other people started arriving and they were remarkably like me. Forty-something, in track pants and t-shirts, no airs and graces. No athleisure or active wear; just a common interest in a thousand-year-old practice.

Those first few sessions of yoga made me feel sick, nauseous, and were far from calming my mind. In fact, I couldn't even do the breathing exercises!

Breathing, for God's sake! I couldn't even breathe properly!

And, as for downward-facing dog, you had to be joking. My spindly little arms could not hold my body up. I was thinking, *this is not for me, what is this yoga stuff?* All I felt like doing was vomiting.

The only thing that kept me going back was my yoga teacher. She honestly looked like she had a halo above her head—an aura? I don't know what you call it but I so wanted to be like that. She was serene, calm, and had a wicked sense of humour. When your yoga class music is Africa by Toto, you have to be on to something good!

I started thinking maybe this yoga stuff could be alright if I stuck it out. I had nothing else on the horizon other than looking down the barrel of twelve months of cancer treatment; anything had to be better than nothing.

I persevered through another four weeks of classes until one day it just came to me. I could do it – it was really making me feel better in my head.

I strangely became quickly addicted to it. I signed up for workshops, added classes, and roped my husband in. I declared that, "Yoga has changed my life." And it has, in more ways than one.

Yoga was my saviour in those few months of chemotherapy treatment, and I started to look forward to my classes more than ever. Yoga has recently become one of the biggest wellness trends in the world and I couldn't be happier. In fact, according to Ray Morgan research in 2016, 1 in 10 Australians do yoga, which has doubled since 2008.

I felt the attraction to the ancient practice and I knew it was changing my perception, my mind, and my sense of calmness.

Yoga is generally recognised as an ancient system of philosophies, principles and practices derived from the Vedic tradition of India and the Himalayas more than 2,500 years ago. It recognizes the multi-dimensional nature of the human person and relates it to the nature and workings of the mind.

There is something strangely addictive about yoga; I would never have believed it. I started to research why it made me feel better. I had such a sense of wellness and peace when I finished class, I couldn't understand how a few pretzel poses could make so much difference to how I was feeling. It was the only exercise I did though my treatment other than walking.

Yoga is a very old practice, as a westerner I had very little knowledge of these ancient practices. I knew few people who practiced yoga and no one really seemed to talk about it. Well, no one I knew. My sister was a convert but because I wasn't in that 'space' I never asked her about why she did it. How did she feel mentally and physically after a class? I had to find out! I had a new purpose, my mind was starting to turn and I could feel the presence of something bigger than me. The universe was sending me a message and I needed to stand up and listen.

"Bring attention to the body." That is the opening statement when we start our yoga classes. The practice of Yoga Nidra, also known as 'psychic sleep', is a deep relaxation technique in yoga. It is by far my favourite part of the classes. You bring attention in a systematic way to different parts of your body, like the top of your head, your face, neck, and then eventually all the way down to your toes, going over every part of your body. It is amazing!

According to the yoga journal yin yoga "is designed to help you sit longer, and more comfortable, in meditation by stretching connective tissues around the joints (mainly the knees, pelvis, sacrum and spine) A passive practice, Yin Yoga involves variations of seated and supine poses typically held for 3 to 5 minutes".

Doing something as simple as a mindful yin yoga practice was a revelation to me. I couldn't believe how calm and in tune with myself I had become. It was unbelievable, how come I had never heard of it? No medical person had mentioned it to me. I guess it wasn't the science of medicine, but I was intrigued.

Well, I went a bit crazy town and bought up books about mindfulness. I wanted to find out as much as I could; being an avid reader I ploughed through these books with the fervour of a madwoman. My absolute favourite books on mindfulness are by Ruby Wax, her take on mindfulness is spot on and hilarious. She has two books, and they are equally fantastic. *Sane New World* and *Frazzled*.

Ruby has a wonderful way of writing for the common person; she is wickedly funny about a serious subject and offers so many gems in her books that resonated with me. Ruby had suffered depression, which led to her studying mindfulness at Oxford. Whilst I wasn't in that academic space, I saw parallels with the feelings I had after my cancer diagnosis.

# CHAPTER 10

I woke up one night covered in sweat; I was so hot I had completely thrown the bed covers on the floor. Oh God, I had a fever. The nurses told me if my temperature rose above thirty-eight degrees then I was to contact the hospital.

I had been so careful not to catch any germs while I was doing chemo, I used hand sanitiser practically ten times a day; I had a big pump pack full of it near the front door so my husband and children could wash their hands with it before they came near me. I developed a phobia of germs, which kept me vigilant. And there I was, lying in bed sweating like crazy, my forehead dripping.

I started to panic; I didn't want to go to the hospital. I couldn't get sick. What about my white blood cell count? What about those neutrophils the nurses keep going on about? All those blood tests before my chemo, surely they would have indicated an infection?

Hang on. I suddenly didn't feel hot anymore. What was going on? The sweating stopped. Maybe I was just a bit anxious. It repeated another two times during the night. In the morning it dawned on me: I was having hot flushes.

Well, that was something I was not prepared for; no one tells you just how quickly chemo shrivels up your ovaries and sends you into early menopause. Good Lord, could it get any worse? Not only did

I have to deal with a breast cancer diagnosis, surgery, and chemo, radiation: now I had to deal with having menopause.

I cried again, cried at the injustice of it all. It hit me hard. I had two beautiful children and I wasn't planning anymore, but the fact that having cancer had now robbed me of my fertility was the last straw. The poison running through my veins was now wreaking havoc with my ovaries.

I found out that day that depending on how old you are, and what type and dosage of chemo you have, your ovaries may or may not recover from this damage.

What? May or may not? What on the earth did that mean? Had I gone into early menopause or not? From what I had read from the Cancer Council literature, it seemed very likely that I had. In fact, if you are over forty when diagnosed, you have a 70-90% chance of going into permanent menopause from chemotherapy.

There were those statistics again, and not in my favour. The whole cancer thing just kept on giving, and giving, and giving. I didn't want any of it.

The menopause on top of a breast cancer diagnosis can be more than a major disruption. It can wreck your sex life, dash hopes of having a baby, trigger mood swings, produce debilitating hot flashes, cause weight gain, drain your energy, worsen aches and pains, bring on jealousy or anger or resentment and leave you feeling anything but yourself. You may find it's these menopausal changes, not the breast cancer or the effects of the treatment that interfere most with your quality of life. Wow. So much to look forward to.

If I could look on the positive side of it, then at least I didn't have to buy pads and tampons anymore. That was one plus, no more periods. I could now go out and buy some more white jeans.

But I couldn't believe I had that to deal with on top of everything else; I felt the weight on my shoulders, when was it going to stop? How much more would I have to endure? It was still early days, how was I going to cope with another twelve months of it? Quite frankly, at that rate, I thought I wouldn't even see the year out; it really was going to kill me, after all.

The hot flushes in the early days were debilitating, I would spontaneously start sweating at any given time; during a meeting at work, in yoga class, travelling on the train, sitting at my desk, cooking, and worst of all, at night-time. I was up out of bed two to three times a night from the sweats, all varying levels of it; sometimes just a red face, sometimes swimming in sweat. I was exhausted from chemo, exhausted from lack of sleep, and exhausted from life. What a nightmare.

Several things happened in my life at that time. My brother announced he was getting married, I signed up to do a ten day trek in the heart of Tuscany (Italy) for Breast Cancer Network Australia (BCNA) and a very good friend of mine who I had lost touch with came back into my life. All three events made me change direction; it was the pivotal change I needed.

## CHAPTER 11

I had finally awoken out of the fog, life was turning on its axis, and I had an opportunity to pull myself out of the rabbit hole. It was happening for a reason, I had no answers just an overwhelming sense that the universe had things in store for me. For the first time in months, I could see the wood for the trees. I had a purpose.

My brother had got engaged on Valentine's Day, one week before my diagnosis, and a lifetime ago in my world. I was super happy for him at the time but recent events had totally eclipsed any thoughts of the newly engaged couple. I thought at least I would have twelve months to contemplate attending a wedding. But guess what my brother said, "We are getting married in May!"

How was I going to attend a family wedding halfway through chemo when no one in my family knew I had breast cancer? Oh shit, game was up and I wasn't ready.

I still cannot really remember how I found out about Breast Cancer Network Australia (BCNA) Trek to Tuscany. I think it may have been the first time I got onto BCNA's website, trying to find information on breast cancer.

*"Congratulations Jane on taking the first step on joining an incredible and inspiring journey with Breast Cancer Network Australia! On this amazing 10-day adventure, you'll journey to the heart of Tuscany, Italy. Trekking over 5 days through picturesque countryside, provincial villages and medieval towns, you will experience all the breathtaking beauty that Tuscany has to offer. Best of all, you'll be raising vital funds to help BCNA support all Australians affected by breast cancer."*

What had I done? I'm hardly an intrepid traveller, I was still doing chemo, and Herceptin and radiation were booked for August. I had told practically no one that I had breast cancer. How was I going to raise $4,000 when no one knew why I would be doing such a trip? Why, all of sudden, was Jane raising money for BCNA? I had paid the non-refundable deposit, I was going, and I had no idea how I was going to do it.

Then along came my friend.

I had missed her, and thought of her often. We had known each other for thirteen years; we were close, we shared secrets, she was my sounding board, and if you think of the definition of a friend, "a person with whom one has a bond of mutual affection", she was all of that and more.

Our relationship soured when she left her job and started her own business. I should have been happy for her, I should have supported her in her new venture, but I didn't. I scorned her positive attitude and bravery for stepping out on her own, and month after month I slowly let her go out of my life. I remember someone saying to me once that people come and go in your life, they are there for a reason and then they go. I thought, well, that is that then, she was meant to be in my life then, but not now. I hadn't seen her for two years.

I was a third of the way through chemo and still had eight treatments to go. I was ticking off each Friday on the calendar as it came around; it was the longest week in my life and the shortest the week in my life. Time had no bearing; just week in week out of going to hospital, visiting the specialists, and having blood tests. When would it all end?

The treatment was relentless but the medical appointments were worse. In one week I would realistically see three doctors and have two to three tests, it was too much. *Way* too much.

Every time I visited one of those people, I was reminded of what happened. Reminded of my cancer. People poked and prodded, there was no dignity, there was no compassion. I was just another person in a long line of cancer patients. It is all so humiliating, exhausting, and I wanted out.

I was treating my hair with kid gloves, and it was hanging in there. The cold cap was working. Four weeks after my first chemo treatment and I still had my long hair. What a miracle, I felt blessed. No one could tell I was having treatment, the most obvious of side effects had eluded me and I couldn't be happier. I still looked like me; I could look in the mirror and see myself, not a cancer patient, which was very reassuring and gave me the confidence to just get on with it. I didn't fit the typical picture of a cancer sufferer. I could hide.

My girlfriends continued to support me in the chemo ward and were starting to become better known by the staff and other patients than me.

"What a great day in the chemo ward, Jane! I had fun! That somehow sounds a tiny bit wrong."

She was right though, a chemo ward is full of the most inspiring people. They are fabulous company and they, of all people, just get it. They are in the same boat as you. In fact, I think everyone should spend a day in a chemotherapy department because it would make most people's problems insignificant. There is nothing like a bit of perspective.

I remember reading somewhere that, 'everyone should get cancer once in their life', because of the life changing experience. I'm not sure I wanted this particular life changing experience, thanks. Why couldn't I have just got sacked or something? That would be life changing. Why did it have to be cancer?

# CHAPTER 12

Every week would pass with different emotions, some weeks I was good, some weeks I was terrified. There was so much in between. I was on a roller coaster and I was mentally exhausted.

It was approaching winter, my favourite time of year. My neighbourhood was full of beautiful English Oaks with leaves the size of your hand. Autumn had brought these beauties floating off their stems into our laneways, streets, and gardens. I loved the crunch under my feet when I went out for my walk. The milder weather and the darker afternoons were an assault on my senses. I loved it.

Except I was looking down the barrel of spending all of autumn and winter in cancer treatment.

As the weather changed, so did my mood. I love the cold weather and I finally found some peace by rugging up in my winter woollies and walking. I would come home from chemo on Friday afternoons and quickly change into my walking shoes and hoodie. The wind and dampness of the air on my face, the smell of the winter roses hanging on the fence, leaves crunching under my feet... I could lose myself in this place and be happy. I could leave my worries behind me for a few hours. It was cathartic.

The inner peace was rising from my heart and I am pretty sure it was because of all those endorphins releasing themselves when I exercised. Why had I not thought of it before? Regular exercise has been proven to reduce stress, it could help me focus on the positives and stop me from getting caught up in the whirlwind of cancer. Previous to that I had come home and sat on the couch after chemo, too emotionally tired to do anything.

I also had to book a flight to Darwin because my brother was getting married. I was only half way through chemo and I had to take a week's break from treatment. It was good and bad; good, because I got two weeks off from treatment but bad, because it put my treatment back a week, so I would finish later than expected. Bummer. Instead of counting down I had to add another week.

But on the bright side, I had some time off from being a cancer patient. How grand! And I got a mini medical holiday in the tropics while the weather back home was cold. Plus, I got to see my family, which is always lovely. I set about booking my flights and contacting my dear friends in Darwin to see if I could stay with them for the weekend.

I had no intention of saying anything about my cancer diagnosis to anyone. I just wanted to be normal, do normal things, go out for dinner, relax, and have a glass of wine and a cigarette. I wanted out of the life I had been living since February. But it dawned on me that I couldn't travel interstate without at least one person knowing about my condition and treatment—that would have been a bit irresponsible of me. If something happened to me, someone had to know.

I decided to send my two friends I was staying with in Darwin an email, letting them know what had been happening in my life. It was the first time I constructed an email about what had happened. It was hard not to ramble on about it, and just state the facts, giving enough information that I didn't have to explain things ten times over.

Afterwards, I used that same email to send to people, once I became more comfortable with my diagnosis and what had been happening in my life.

Those friends had been in Bali too, when we celebrated my dad's 70th birthday, and were as unaware as the rest of my family. I dearly wanted to tell them, I have known my girlfriend for twenty-three years. She is very special to me and has had experience with cancer, through her husband who had been treated and made a full recovery. She knew what it was like from the outside looking in. She knew how devastating it could be for the person to deal with a diagnosis and treatment. I was OK with telling them, I knew I had to.

It felt really wonderful to share my news with my friends. The night I arrived in Darwin we sat on their balcony until 2am in the morning, just talking, and it felt good to let it all out.

I had a favour to ask of my girlfriend. My hair, by that stage, was very fragile from the cold cap treatment and I couldn't cut it. I wanted to look as normal as possible—that point was imperative.

"Now, hair—Jane how long have you known me? Is styling hair my thing? No. However you may be surprised to learn I have a mini hair dryer that works and blows a lot of air, plus a hair straightening thing, but not GDH—GHD—you know what. That's about it. No brush—seriously. I'm happy to give it a crack but I'm warning you... I'd suggest you ask your sister to come around but I don't know if you've told your family yet. Otherwise, it's salon time, Janey-Jane!"

She made me laugh. It made me realise just how crazy my life had become, here I was worried about my hair. My hair, of all things! I have never been a person to worry about having great hair. I too didn't own a decent hair brush. As it turned out, I did my own hair with my girlfriend double-checking the back of my head to make sure none of my slightly bald patches were showing.

I look back on those photos now, and I am totally in awe of the fact I look half decent and my hair is perfect! Job well done!

Being in the tropics again took me back to being in Bali when I felt like I was living a normal life. No hospital appointments, no doctors and specialist appointments, a 'medical holiday'—how wonderful. It rejuvenated me.

My brother's wedding was beautiful, and as we arrived at the reception, the sun was starting to set over the Darwin Harbour. It sizzled on the horizon and was calming and reassuring to be seeing nature in all its glory.

What a beautiful spot. Palm trees, frangipanis, tropical paradise. I was far away from what my life had become. I soaked it in, and for the first time in a while I felt happy. As I sat watching the sun set, I poured myself a glass of wine and thought, I will get through this. I will be OK. I just had to trust it too shall pass, and focus on living one day at a time.

A sense of relief passed over me; I could see myself in the future, I could see myself happy.

As the night passed with good food, good wine, and good company, the night time air had got quite humid. I kicked my shoes off under the table because my feet had swollen in the heat. I got up to go the toilet, which was around the back of the building, and as I came out I tripped on my own long flowing pants and sent myself crashing on the pavers below. Of course as falls go, it all happened in slow motion. I tripped, tried to push upright again, and kept falling forward until my right big toe and knee took the brunt of my fall.

Oh God, there was blood pouring out of my toe. I quickly picked myself up and rushed back into the bathroom, where I propped myself up on the bench and put my foot under the running water. Blood was everywhere. All over the basin; it was coming out of my knee, too.

Oh God, it was not something I had even thought about. What happens when you cut yourself while you are on chemo? Did I have to go to the hospital? I didn't even have a band aid on me, let alone bandages to cover it up. I had no choice after the blood had subsided but to go back to the table and ask my sister whether she had any band aids. She did, thankfully, and said what a silly duffer I'd been while she patched up my knee and toe.

My head was swirling with worries of getting an infection; it was not the time to announce to my family I had cancer.

As I hobbled back to the table, I had probably gone a bit white and was met with reassurances like, "Don't worry, it will be fine, it's just a bit of skin you've taken off."

Normally I would have laughed it off, too. I can be clumsy at the best of times, but it couldn't have been worse timing. I had to take the best care of myself during chemo and scrapping the skin off your toe and knee wasn't ideal. God, I am a klutz.

When I returned to my friend's apartment, I jumped straight in the shower to wash out the wounds and get rid of the insect repellent I had sprayed all over me in the attempt to not get bitten by mosquitoes (it didn't work, I was also itching like crazy). I was starting to panic. Maybe I should have gone to the hospital? But then I would have had to explain my whole story and I wasn't prepared for that, I didn't want to go through it. What a drag.

I decided to cover the open wounds in Betadine, patch them up with band-aids, and leave them until I got home – and that was what I did. With no help from my girlfriend, who was gagging from the sight of the skin missing from my toe.

The rest of the weekend passed without incident and too soon I was on my way home, back to the reality of life. It was so lovely to have the break, to rejuvenate after weeks of chemotherapy, my body needed it. I wished I never had to go back to the oncology ward, but alas no, my next treatment was in four days' time. My toe and knee recovered well. I did go to my GP the day after I arrived back, and he said, "You probably should have gone to the hospital."

## CHAPTER 13

Number six chemo done, half way there. What a milestone. I was celebrating the little things. One week at a time, that was the only way to tackle it. My girlfriends would send me little snippets of positivity, which I loved and relished at the time. There had to be something positive to come out of all of this. My favourite from this time was, "Surround yourself with people who make you hungry for life, touch your heart and nourish your soul." Such a beautiful sentiment.

I had given my mum tickets to an exhibition of costumes from a drama series on television for Mother's Day, which included afternoon tea. It was easier to give my parents 'experiences', they didn't need anything, and my mum had enjoyed that particular television series so it was a good choice.

I gave her two tickets and fully intended for my dad to accompany her. But dad didn't want to go so she asked if I would like to. Not really. I had to be careful not be out and about too much where I could catch some sort of bug that would compromise my immune system. I had been so careful and I didn't want to take unnecessary risks. But my mum didn't know I had breast cancer, let alone being pumped full of poison every week. I wasn't ready to tell her, so I agreed to go.

Sundays were my worst day post-treatment. Fridays I was as high as a kite on steroids. Saturdays I was still OK as the chemo hadn't quite kicked in, but by Sunday I always felt like I had been hit by a bus. I very rarely organised anything for a Sunday. It was my day to lie on the sofa, read, and generally do very little.

I found that I started to rally by Tuesday and then Wednesday and Thursday were good until I was hit again on Fridays. I knew the cycle well, it was very predictable, and I could organise my week around it. How crap that my life had become a scheduled succession of medical and hospital appointments, with my weekends reduced to being a hermit.

At least it wasn't summer—that was a blessing—I was happy to be indoors all rugged up.

But Mum decided that Sunday would be a good day to go to the exhibition and I couldn't say anything. The weather had turned bitterly cold and I took extra care to rug up and wear six layers of clothes. It would have been OK any other time, but on the hour, every hour, I was sweating like a person in tropical climates, not mid-winter in Melbourne. I was constantly stripping clothes on and off, that in itself was exhausting. When Mum and I sat down for afternoon tea, she said quite concerningly that she wanted to talk to me about menopause. Oh, great.

"You know, I got early menopause. I was only forty-two."

I knew. But it was different for me. Not only was I older than Mum at forty-seven, my menopause was chemically induced. It wasn't normal menopause. I really didn't want to have that whole conversation; I was tired, feeling rather shady, and sweating profusely under my jacket. I was very self-conscious, too. My eyebrows had started thinning, I had lost a chunk of eyelashes on the corner of my right eye, and my hair was brittle and dry.

I didn't want anyone getting too close to me otherwise there were too many questions. I put on a brave face in front of my mum in the 1950's inspired tea rooms – yet I felt about as old and haggard as the surroundings.

*Tuscany Trek*

*"Your Journey is Beginning"*

# CHAPTER 14

Oops, there I go again, I had totally forgotten to start fundraising!

I put that thought on the back-burner for another month or so, until I reached week eleven of my chemotherapy. One more treatment and I was done with chemo. I cannot tell you how good that felt; I was over the moon. All that counting down for the last thirteen weeks and I was nearly there.

I had endured the scalp cooling every week and was ecstatic that my hair had not fallen out. I was one of the 60% it had worked for. I may not have had statistics on my side with my diagnosis or menopause, but the scalp cooling was in my favour.

By all intents and purposes, I did not 'look' like a cancer patient. I could hide my diagnosis and I was very happy about that. It meant I could go to work every day, go to yoga, go shopping, and see my family, with no one any the wiser. I was in control of how I looked to everyone out there, which was a huge relief; I had gotten away with it. No one suspected anything. I could deal with it myself with only my small circle of friends. I was alright.

I still felt like I was climbing Everest, but I was getting closer to the top, on my way to the other side.

My last day of chemo was the best day ever!

I was counting down big time. After weeks of ticking off the calendar, there I was at the very last day. I could not have been happier. The last three months may have gone fast for everyone else, but it was the slowest three months for me.

The scalp cooling had made my chemo sessions quite the marathon. If I had just had chemo, I would have been in and out in three hours. Each of my visits were at least five hours.

Going to the toilet was a huge problem. Not only was I hooked up to an IV, I was hooked up to two pipes on the scalp cooling machine which had to be disconnected to move anywhere. Every time I needed to go to the toilet, I would have to call the nurses so that I could be disconnected. Which, of course, caused the cap to not be at the correct temperature so I had to be pretty quick, otherwise my scalp would get warmer and I so did not want that. I was trying to keep my hair.

Along with having to drink plenty of water while you have chemo, they also pump saline through the IV, which doubles the dose of fluid. I used to sit in the chair absolutely busting to go to the toilet and I would only move if I couldn't hold it in anymore. I got pretty good at it; I got it down to one toilet visit per session. I seriously wanted to use an adult nappy because I hated the whole toilet thing. I would have to sometimes go out into the hospital corridor to go to the toilet and that was embarrassing enough. Let alone having to manage pipes like out of control octopus legs, grappling with the toilet door—all while trying not to pull out my IV. It was a complete nightmare. I started getting anxious about going to the toilet. For God's sake! I wish I had used the nappies.

I will not miss that cap, no matter how much I might have looked like I was competing in the Olympics; I never want to wear one again. I took a few photos of me in the cumbersome contraption—they are hilarious to look back at now—but at the time it was mixed blessings. Miraculous that the strange machine saved my hair, but

I would prefer not to have needed it at all. Even after all those months, I could not believe I was in that predicament, still having to subject myself to more torture. It really boggles the mind. But, the ugly and uncomfortable cap was worth it.

I wore a crown on my last day of chemo.

My girlfriend said, "Awesome, the crowns suits you; you should have been royalty, Jane."

I felt pretty regal that day. I was the star of the show, my last chemo day, it seems crazy but I was relieved beyond belief. I had put my crown on and I was walking, walking straight out of day oncology and never going back.

I had made it through twelve rounds of weekly chemotherapy and had gotten through it relatively unscathed. Someone was looking after me. Besides having diarrhoea for three months, fatigue, discoloured nails, and constant bloody noses, I was feeling OK. My hair had hung on for dear life and my body had coped well. I had a lot to be thankful for.

I'm glad I never read the reams of paper on side effects; I think if I had read them, I would have been concentrating on the negatives and not concentrating on the positives. I had started to be very aware of my thoughts by that stage and it was important to me to focus on all the good things in my life. I had 'graduated' from chemo. And I was looking forward to doing a proper poo.

Even from a young age I immersed myself in books as often as I could. Enid Blyton was my favourite. I truly believed there was a Faraway tree with magical folk. I loved reading about Moonface, Silky and the Saucepan Man. I could escape into that world whenever I wanted. I had a love for the world of books and my imagination ran wild. I have never lost that feeling, being immersed in words. I will read about anything; botany, history, travel writing, religion, anything. My favourite authors now are Elizabeth Gilbert and Bill Bryson; I have read their books countless times.

I scour school fetes, church fairs, charity shops, and local bookstores for the next fix. I had purpose built bookshelves at home to house my ever-growing library of books. I never give them away, I couldn't bear to part with them. I have read every book on my shelves at least once, in some cases seven-eight times. I have my favourites that I re-read at least once every two years. Besides, if I didn't enjoy reading, I don't think I would want to write.

*Why People Fail* by Siimon Reynolds, was not a book I had read more than once. In fact I had bought it and only skimmed over the chapters, I didn't remember one bit of the book. I can't tell you why that one particular book found me. I have no answer as to why I felt compelled to pull it off my bookshelf. The front of the book hooks the reader into wanting to find out what the sixteen principles are that will change your life.

Wow! That sounded like either a miracle or just another self-help book to me. But I had grabbed it off the shelf so that had to mean something.

I remember this author from the eighties. He was an advertising man, one of Australia's youngest self-made millionaires, but somehow all I can remember about him was that his first name had two 'i's.

No matter, because there I was taking his book down five years after buying it, looking inside for a message. Something that would ease my pain, something that would help me heal my mind. I was looking everywhere by that point. My yoga had helped a lot but I wanted to learn more about how I could lift myself out of the fog, how I could keep going. How was I going to get through this?

I only needed to read the first chapter, called Unclear Purpose, to get to my 'ah-ha' moment.

## CHAPTER 15

"What is my life purpose?"

I didn't want my current life anymore, it was dreadful. It was not who I was, I was a stranger in my own mind. I needed to start looking from the inside out; I needed to get out of the prison I was in.

"What is my life purpose?" I asked myself again. "I want to be a higher spiritual person, and I want to help people."

That is what I wrote on the first page of my journal. I had no idea how I was going to do it, but those words resonated with me and I started writing. My husband and children had given me a diary for Mother's Day. It was a gratitude diary. I remember thinking at the time there was nothing to be grateful for.

I had cancer, and on Mother's Day I underwent my fourth chemo treatment—still looking down the barrel of months of truly dreadful treatment. I didn't feel grateful at all, in fact I was the opposite; ungrateful and unappreciative of everything at that point. I put that little book in my bedside drawer and promptly forgot about it.

According to Siimon's book I needed to write things down. I needed to be in the moment. To find what things boosted my happiness. So what could I be doing to boost my happiness? I had to give it a go – I thought this sounded easy enough. I could do this. I had to try as much as possible to see the good in everything. OK, I got that. So I simply needed to start my own happiness habit.

Alright then, next to practice gratitude. This was a new concept to me but one that seemed to be gaining traction over the last few years. Be grateful and that means being grateful for everything in your life, even the little things.

I pulled that little book out of the bedside drawer, dusted it off, and began my daily practice of writing. I just wrote scribble to begin with, anything about how I was feeling. It was cathartic, and it didn't matter what it was. I would write down lyrics from songs that I heard on the radio, I would write about my day, what had made me happy during that particular day and why. I would write about the weather, I would write about people in my life.

But the one thing I didn't write about was cancer. That was the no-go zone. "Count your blessings." That was the message. So I could only write about the good things in my day, the things that I was grateful for. At the end of the day I would re-read my words and feel a real sense of relief. It reaffirmed that focusing on the good things was making me feel better.

There are of course countless books, articles, lectures, and courses on how to be happy, you can take your pick. You know it is your natural state, to be happy. I knew it too. But when you are blindsided by a cancer diagnosis, you don't know how to be happy. I didn't have a clue. My happiness had gone on holiday and it was looking more and more permanent. I would lie awake at night trying to see sense in my predicament. I had received the worst news of my life, it was more than just a difficult time. I was in shock and petrified. I had never felt like that before. Happy? You had to be joking!

When difficult times befall you, it is hard to admit to yourself that the life that you had, the life you had worked hard to create, wasn't there anymore and not only that, it was falling apart.

Writing about what was good in my life started changing my perspective. Not straight away, but day in day out I would write a few words. I used to sit there, pen poised, and struggle to think of something positive to write. I really had to try, try and think of the best things that had happened in my day. That was sad to me, it was sad that I felt I had nothing to be grateful for.

It took quite a lot of time to write anything on those pages. The first few weeks, I wrote about my children mainly, because they make me happy. I love them with all my heart. They had no idea what was going on in my head, life was business as usual for them. They both celebrated birthdays during my chemo. They were blissfully unaware and that made me happy. I didn't want them to be sad and miss out on all their milestones because of me.

# CHAPTER 16

Day by day I found more things to be happy and grateful for—just little things. I felt blessed I had such wonderful friends who would accompany me to chemo. I was happy my husband cooked dinner and did the laundry. I was happy when it rained. Anything and everything—it didn't matter what. The fact I was writing it down was enough.

I guess a diary is writing to yourself, though I had never really thought about the practice much. I never kept a diary as a child. I used to write things down but not in the sense of a 'dear diary', although I remember it being popular in the 80's. Writing about how you feel was pretty foreign to me; I thought it was a bit silly. I wasn't always great at remembering to do the daily task but as I started to become more aware of how I was changing, I began to crave writing and sending myself little notes and inspirations. I didn't want to miss a day and after a while, it became part of my daily ritual.

I started to change the story I was telling myself. Refocusing on the belief I was going to be absolutely fine, I was going to recover from treatment, I was going to rid my body of cancer and I was never going to get it back. Full stop.

All of those thoughts that circled in my head about cancer were starting to become less noisy. Countless articles and literature on cancer tell you, 'you are not alone', which is a strange concept to me. I was alone, there was only me, I was the only one going through it, I could be nobody else. I had to look after me, just me, my own thoughts.

I wasn't alone as such, I had a small support team of other people but in my mind, I was the only one who could help me. It didn't matter what they said, they could never know what it was like to be me. My inner self, my inner peace, had to recognise my dark thoughts were not me.

Your thought are like clouds, they come and go all day and some are good, some not so good, but they are not you. That was a revelation, a true revelation. I am not my thoughts, my thoughts are not me. What freedom I was experiencing, a freedom from my own thoughts.

I started to look for articles about thankfulness. I happened across an article that said being grateful is actually good for your health.

When it comes to managing our well-being we are told to count our blessings. Focusing on the positive and the good things in our life can bring a range of benefits, including increased well-being and reduced depression.

I can say first hand I felt those benefits; I was slowly coming out of the fog by writing. Who would have guessed? It became easy for me to see the positive things in my life. I still had bad days but they were starting to be overridden by the good days; a change I thought would never happen.

I took to writing a gratitude list every day.

This is my list of things I am grateful for (2016 edition):
1. The love, generosity, and patience of my family and friends

and how lucky I am to have you all in my life
2. My furry friends for entertaining me while I was high on steroids and couldn't sleep
3. The smell of frangipani flowers, that smell is heaven on earth
4. Nurses, they are all angels
5. Turmeric lattes, I have become addicted to them
6. Yoga, my new love
7. Jamie Oliver's 30 minute meals. It's the best cookbook ever
8. My job, for letting me take the time off I needed to have treatment
9. OPI nail varnish (at least my nails looked good during chemo)
10. Blueberries
11. UGG Boots, preferred footwear for home, hospital, and going to yoga
12. Bali, paradise on earth
13. Sauvignon Blanc (at least I could have a glass of wine during chemo)
14. My gift of health
15. My hair, for not falling out
16. Elizabeth Gilbert, her books are my favourite
17. Art galleries and museums the world over, I am a sucker for a beautiful painting
18. BCNA
19. The view from our apartment roof terrace in New York
20. My beautiful husband and children. They are my everything.

## CHAPTER 17

I had always been a little bit spiritual, not a lot, but I loved reading my horoscopes, occasionally had my tarot cards read, and genuinely believe I had an angel looking over me. My angel was always there and I would sometimes talk to her and thank her for looking after me and my family.

I am by no stretch of the imagination new age or religious, I have no opinion on any 'god' but I do believe we are all part of the spiritual universe. Not that I ever thought about it much until then. The cancer diagnosis made me rethink practically everything in my life. I had recently read, "What if the worst day of your life is actually the best day of your life, you just can't see it?"

That statement made me cry.

I realised right then, being diagnosed with breast cancer was the best day of my life. Regardless of how I had been thinking previously, it happened for a reason and I needed to take it as a sign. A sign there is something else for me to do.

I knew what it was; I wanted to help people. I wanted to help people get through the truly terrifying news they have cancer. I wanted to help people get through the maze that was this awful disease and how to cope. I knew first-hand how truly devastating it is, the feeling of helplessness, the suicidal thoughts, the reassurance that everything will be alright, that it too shall pass.

Except, how was I going to do that?

## CHAPTER 18

*"We are delighted to have you as part of our BCNA Tuscany Trek in 2017! It takes a special kind of person to take on a challenge like this and I genuinely look forward to working with you over the coming months to assist you with your fundraising and training for this exciting adventure!"*

Oh. I had again completely forgotten I signed up for a trek! Oops.

I had gone on to BCNA's website once to sign up for the trek. I thought it best to have another look. As I navigated around BCNA's website I realised that the wad of books in the pink bag the Breast Care Nurse had left me at the hospital was a, 'My Journey Kit' from BCNA.

I have to say right now, I loathe the word 'journey'. It either conjures up Frodo and his magic ring travelling through Middle Earth, or an X Factor contestant. Neither one relates to me and my cancer diagnosis. It was not a ticket to anywhere; I was not going on a journey!

I had read an article about Emily McDowell; she is a Los Angeles based designer who had stage three Hodgkin's Lymphoma. She said during her treatment that many of my close friends and family members disappeared because they didn't know what to say, or said the absolute wrong thing.

Emily launched a series of Empathy Cards after her experience and she has some fantastic cards that people can give someone who is going through cancer.

On the subject of what not to say to someone who has had cancer; it is a minefield. I think there are three schools of thought. The person who says nothing, the person who says all the wrong things, and the person who is super supportive and knows exactly what to say. I had a mixture of all.

The person who says nothing is a hard one, especially when it is a close family member.

I know everyone deals with a cancer diagnosis differently; I sure have over the years. But when you tell people you have cancer, you expect people would be at least compassionate, kind, and possibly offer help. Even if that just meant making a meal, or offering to do the grocery shopping. I really shouldn't have had any expectation, as I was only disappointed. It was a huge revelation that some people would turn this around to be about them and not me.

I found it difficult to begin with. I think I expected my family especially, to be the most supportive, the most compassionate, the most likely to offer up assistance. What I found was the people you least expected would help were the ones who did, and vice versa.

It was such an insight to me. I had not considered certain people wouldn't be there for me. I had in the past gone out of my way to help, offered support financially and emotionally, to many people in my life and when I needed the support they were not there. It was devastating at the time, but I realised they had always been like that; I had just never seen it.

Existentially people only care about themselves. It is not a bad thing as it is self-preservation. Look after yourself because you are the only one you have. Nonetheless, I felt abandoned by the very people I thought were going to always be there for me. That was life changing in more ways than one.

But I was self-preserving, too. I understood I needed to think of myself first and foremost.

I believe some people thought when I didn't tell them about my diagnosis it meant I didn't need their love and support. That is OK, I needed to extend the peace pipe. I needed to forgive the people who didn't think being there for me was an option.

Many people really don't know what to say. I have been guilty of this myself in the past, especially when someone has lost a friend or family member. You want to help, to say the right things, but somehow it comes out all wrong. I get tongue twisted and end up saying something completely inappropriate like, "I don't know what to say." How original of me. I just sounded like an idiot.

I, too, had the same conversation with people but I was OK with it because I wouldn't know what to say to me either. In fact, I was talking to myself all the time and I wasn't even saying the right things.

I cannot say I was ever really offended by what people said, except the one time someone said to me, "You deserve to get cancer because you smoke." Gee, thanks. No one deserves to get cancer regardless of their life style decisions. It was a very cruel thing to say.

Back to the BCNA website.

Well, it has a lot of information. I cherry picked what I wanted to know about, which in my case was still very little, but I was drawn to their online network. It was launched in 2010 and is a network to connect Australians affected by breast cancer. I started to read some of the posts and, quite frankly, started crying.

The stories were mostly quite depressing. I had to stop. It wasn't helping. Reading other people's experiences only highlighted that I was going through the same thing, with all of the same emotions. It was too raw at that stage, I still had ten months of treatment to go, and my 'happiness boosters' were failing.

I decided to have a good look at what this trek was all about instead. I had signed up for something I knew very little about, I truly said yes on a whim and now was facing the harsh reality of whether I would be able to do it or not. What was the adventure? It was ten days "trekking through the heart of picture perfect Tuscany, across rolling hills and woodland and provincial towns."

Oh, that sounded quite nice, really. I had heard of other people doing the walk and they raved about it. I could do this, I wanted to help people, I wanted to give something back—that was my new life purpose. "Your fundraising will change lives," was what the brochure said. Well, it was for me then.

I spent some more time looking at BCNA's Online Network, and realised from reading through all the posts that there was a common thread; these people were terrified, they needed reassurance, they need to know they were not alone. They needed to hear from other people who had gone through the same things they were experiencing.

Some of the posts were so depressing, I could feel their anxiety and desperation in their written words, it was soul destroying. I couldn't help but wonder what sort of care they were receiving from the medical professionals who let cancer patients go home and not tell them anything. Who let them wait for weeks in limbo about their results. Why were they having to contact strangers on a website to voice their concerns? And hope someone out there could be a shining light, and relate to what they were feeling right then. Sometimes these posts were 3am in the morning.

My heart went out to these people, it is the most devastating news to receive and these people were scared and sometimes alone, very alone. Some members had watched their own mother's, sisters, and aunts die from breast cancer. They were terrified they would be falling to the same outcome. Some of their stories were truly awful reading, so immensely sad and tragic.

The members who answered were terrific really, they were sometimes years' down the track of diagnosis and treatment, and offered wonderful support through the website. Each new member who received an answer to their posts was so appreciative of the online support. It was heart-warming.

"I feel more positive knowing that you can learn a lot from other people's journeys. One day at a time..." was what one member wrote.

There are also some hilarious stories that make you smile and giggle. Those people got it, they had been through it too.

I realised then there was a lot that I could do, I was one of them too, I was a breast cancer warrior and I wanted to help. I could help people by doing the Tuscany walk for BCNA and I could help people by writing my own story. If I could help just one person, then I would have achieved something.

I knew I had to start fundraising. I had received several emails like, "The countdown to your trek has begun!" and, "Friday fundraising tips." I had to get on with it, but how?

I still hadn't told my parents, my siblings, my work colleagues. The list of people was endless, was I ready to let everyone know? I didn't want to have to repeat myself one hundred times over, I had lots to think about and sometimes 'retelling' the story is tiring when all you want is normal times and conversations. It was a big step to decide to tell everyone.

I knew that it was time to draw on the love and support of the people around me. I was ready. I knew it was time to draw on the love and support of the people around me. I was ready.

My husband wrote my Facebook post. We agreed it was better to come from him. I was happy he could write down what needed to be said and having his perspective on it was cathartic for him too, as he had been the main support person in that chapter of our lives. It just seemed better and more personal.

My aim was not just to let everyone know, but to use my news to spur people into donating to a very worthy cause. It had a very personal slant on it now; I was the one it affected. I was very well aware it was a scatter approach; I knew some people in my family would be upset I didn't tell them personally. I had to do it my way, it was self-preservation, and to this day I do not regret telling my family and friends on Facebook and email.

This was my Facebook post, as written by my husband.

"Hey there everyone.
Here's hoping you and your loved ones are happy and healthy.
You may or may not be aware of recent events in our world. So here it is just in case.
In February of this year (2016) Jane was diagnosed with Stage 2 Breast Cancer. This was a shock especially given her age (under 50) and the speed of the tumour growth.
Jane wanted to approach this issue privately until she was ready to let people know. And now is the time.
To date Jane has:
1. had surgery to remove the tumour and one lymph node.
2. has completed (endured?) 13 weeks of chemotherapy. Every Friday plugged into an IV drip for up to 3 hours. However, is extremely grateful for new 'scalp cooling' technology, which essentially enabled her to keep the majority of her hair (it did thin out, but if you did not know, then you would not have noticed).
3. Will have completed three weeks of radiation therapy, which

will happen every workday for a total of 16 sessions.

4. Has 9 more months of additional 'biological' therapy, and then 5 years of taking a pill!

At the end of all this, there are still no guarantee that it won't return. But by going through the treatment plan the odds are stacked in her favour as much as is possible with today's technology and available medicines.

So what have we learnt from all of this?

i) Jane's type of breast cancer was 100% random. Not genetic, and is not inherited like some other types of breast cancer. So for Jane, it was just pure bad luck. Like many women, 1 in 8 will get breast cancer. These are pretty shitty odds.

ii) Breast cancer can't be prevented.

iii) Breast cancer can occur at ANY age, not just when you're over 50.

iv) Early detection gives you the best possible outcome, and the least invasive treatment.

v) There is no 'standard' breast cancer. There are many, many variations and each with different outcome expectations and treatment plans.

vi) Jane was extremely grateful for scalp cooling technology. This can't be understated in any way. This amazing technology (although uncomfortable and at times painful) enabled Jane to keep this a private process until she was ready to let others know. One of the biggest challenges facing women going through breast cancer treatment is the indignity they feel when they lose their hair. At that stage it is very public and there is no 'hiding' it. In Melbourne only 3 hospitals offer scalp cooling technology, and we were so fortunate that the Epworth in Box Hill (5 minutes from where we live) had one.

vii) Spend just a few days in an oncology ward and talk to some of the women (and men) there and you feel extremely humbled by their positive nature, vibrancy and desire to beat this awful disease.

viii) Nurses are unsung heroes!

ix) Ask lots and lots of questions from your specialists and be prepared to stick up for how you want your treatment to be. One size does not fit all, and everyone should be respected for their right to be treated the way they want to be treated. If you want or need to work during treatment, then ensure your treatment plan works in with your schedule. Your mental health is as important as your physical health.

x) Get moving. Just because you're being treated doesn't mean you should sit around. Recent research shows exercise is an important part of ensuring the treatment goes well. Move every day. Even if it's simply walking for 30-40 minutes.

xi) Get a cold press juicer and start juicing. Include lots of beetroot and ginger.

So, the purpose of this post is twofold.

1. Share this post.

Hopefully you can share this post and let as many women you know about the need to get regular check-ups. And not wait until they're 50 to do so. If Jane had waited until she was 50 it would have been too late!

2. Raise Money

Jane is now dedicated to raise money for Breast Cancer Network Australia (BCNA).

She is going on a self-funded trip to do a Tuscany Walk.

What this means is that the money raised does not pay for the trip. That is paid by us. But the walk is to raise awareness and funds for Breast Cancer.

Jane has a target of $4,000.00 to raise.

So if you are able to contribute any amount at all to this great cause then below is a link to the donation page. Any support would be greatly appreciated and we know first-hand how the funds will be used and the benefit that Australians that are newly diagnosed with breast cancer receive from BCNA.

So, if you are able to provide any support to this amazing cause that affects 1 in 8 women then here's a link to the website ..."

OK, it was out there, and it didn't take long for a tide of responses, phone calls, email, and comments. I was totally blown away with how people were responding to my news. I realised very quickly I had underestimated how much I needed the support of my family and friends.

My cousin wrote the following after hearing of my diagnosis, "Deep breath! That's for sure. I'm still in shock, I am so relieved and happy that you are on the mend and you are going to be okay! I understand you needed space to get your head around this and to recover. Thank you for sharing this news with us. This news has certainly grounded me and made me realise how precious family and our lives are and the day to day issues we encounter and forget that they are not worth worrying about. You are a brave, wonderful and beautiful woman, I am so proud of you."

And another from my niece, "That's a great attitude to have. I mean, I know it is awful, but in a weird sort of way it is sort of a blessing. As you said, it forces you to focus on what really matters, to spend time with those you love and do what makes you happy. Some people don't get that sort of wakeup call until they are much older and many opportunities have already passed them by. So, in that sense, the positive to take I suppose is that you are young, you have people who love you, you have a beautiful family, and it makes you really step back, take stock and appreciate the important things. I know it probably doesn't feel that way when you are in the thick of it, but I guess it's good to try and take positives out of it where you can. You are very loved."

"Thank you for being super strong and positive, for sticking a finger up and fighting back."

I had to be very selective about who I allowed on my 'support team' in the early days. Each of my family members and friends are very close to my heart. But, the reality is not all of them are the best listeners and confidants, especially as you enter what is one of the most challenging times of your life.

Who can you truly rely on to be there in your darkest hour? It was a massive revelation to me that I couldn't rely on some of my closest family. I didn't feel that I could divulge my diagnosis of cancer to the very people who consistently imposed their own health views on me. It wasn't a competition about who was the sickest, or who deserved more compassion. I needed people who would have my own interests at heart, not theirs. It was my path and mine alone. It was not about anyone else's health concerns, health history, or niggling wellness issues. Sometimes their attitudes were overly negative and 'doom and gloom'; I had to stay away from them. They were energy-drainers, and I needed people who were optimistic, positive, and truly cared about what was happening.

In the first week of posting my news on Facebook, I raised an amazing $3,265. I was totally blown away. I was changing people's lives, my family and friends were changing people's lives, including my own. I was bringing happiness to others people through fundraising, and someone out there would benefit from the money I raised. I will never know who they are but I felt profound pride in the fact the very people I read about in the online forum were the people I was helping, and I couldn't have been happier.

$30 - gives women diagnosed with breast cancer a copy of The

Beacon magazine, BCNA's free national magazine for women with breast cancer and their families.

$55 - provides a woman newly diagnosed with a 'My Journey Kit', BCNA's free, comprehensive information resource that offers easy to understand information about treatment and the 'next steps'.

$200 - allows one woman diagnosed with breast cancer to attend a free community information forum with her partner, family or carer.

Members of my husband's family had been so generous with the donations, and written me the most beautiful emails and messages. I couldn't believe it. It cemented in my mind that I had done the right thing by signing up for this fantastic challenge, and telling people my news was a relief. Now it was out in the open, I felt like a weight was off my shoulders.

I don't use Messenger very much, but after my Facebook post I received a message from my absent friend. The friend I had pushed out of my life. "Anything I can do, let me know (would have done sooner if I'd known, but totally get not going public, I wouldn't either!) Keep on kicking ass!"

I was blown away. I hadn't heard from her in two years, I missed her and I couldn't believe that this is what brought us back together—me getting breast cancer. I had missed her friendship, I felt like it was meant to be, our lives were supposed to reconnect again. She was still very much the positive person. I missed her cheery take on the world and I finally realised she was exactly what I need in my life.

# CHAPTER 19

We met years before. We were similar ages and we did the same job. We had a lot in common. Over the years we worked together several times in different businesses and used our lunch breaks and close proximity to each other in the office to talk, gossip, and share hints and tips; a friendship by any other description. She has a very dry sense of humour and I loved her casual approach to life.

When she left her job, I was sad to see her go. Her desk was empty and I couldn't see her everyday like I used to. No more walking through the park for a coffee at lunchtime. I was lost without her.

We kept in touch for a while by email but she had started her own business and I felt annoyed by her positivity and it was all a bit too evangelistic for my liking. All this power of positive thinking stuff—I pooh-poohed it really. I thought it was a bit of a crock. I didn't understand it and I really couldn't be bothered being a part of it either. Her Facebook statuses would pop up on my phone with all this self-help stuff and I used to ignore it. I even started to disengage, so I wouldn't receive them. After that, I just didn't keep in contact. I let the friendship slide, and years of wonderful times, memories, and happiness just disappeared.

We made plans to catch up for lunch a few weeks later. I was really looking forward to seeing her.

It had been an exhausting few weeks just fielding the questions, the concerns, and comments. I received so many messages from people which was incredibly lovely but some were just depressing. I am not sad I got cancer—actually I'm happy I did, it's changed my life. The focus really seemed to be on the negative, so I had to stop that dead in its tracks. I had been there, on the edge of that negative void. Instead, I only wanted to hear the positive stories, and surround myself with positive people who would buoy me and boost my morale. Yes, cancer sucks, but I wanted something good to come out of something bad.

I was really more upbeat after releasing my news to the world, I was buoyed with enthusiasm, I had been practicing yoga for quite some time and it was really making my mind feel calm and clear. I was devouring books on mindfulness. I felt light-hearted and my happiness boosters were on full throttle.

# CHAPTER 20

Life was staring to come back to something that resembled normality, my head space had changed and I was able to see that my thoughts were just that, thoughts: and they can be changed. I love the saying from Louise Hay about it is safe to look within. I felt safe to trust my own instincts, trust my own thoughts and feelings. It was acceptance. I was now able to focus on my recovery.

I still had radiotherapy to complete, so I wasn't quite there yet. By the end of August, I would finally be through the worst of it, and only had Herceptin to continue for the next nine months. I could see some light at the end of the tunnel.

Just like the clouds that come and go, so do storms. I was on the verge of another storm front, and nothing could shake it. I started to become very anxious again. It was the impending radiotherapy treatment; I really was starting to fear it.

My mind had wandered back into familiar territory and it wasn't about to let go yet. My head was spinning and my terror of hospitals was raising its ugly head again. I really thought I was OK, I could handle this, I now had some armour to protect me. I had been a student of yoga for quite some time, I was practicing mindfulness, I was cathartically writing. I had this, I was in control.

But I wasn't.

I expected the wonderful support and compassion I received at my oncology ward throughout my chemotherapy treatment to be the same for radiotherapy. I had high expectations of the care I would receive; I had no reason to think otherwise. It could not have been further from the truth.

My first visit to the radiotherapy department soon made me realise it wasn't going to be the same as my oncology experience. The radiotherapy department is in the bowels of the hospital, it is a dark and dank place, devoid of light and quite frankly frightening and depressing. Not even the pot plant I spotted on the shelf was surviving; its leaves were all curled like it had given up. I got the shock of my life, it was truly awful, it looked like something out of 'one flew over the cuckoo's nest'.

You don't just walk into a radiotherapy unit, you have to check in (and I don't mean like a hotel). You have your photo taken and sign your life away. It is really quite impersonal. A big desk separates you from the staff, and you sit there until someone comes to lead you into the dudgeon. It happened on every visit. No friendly chitchat, no eye contact, no nothing.

I think back now and wonder if I was just fed up at that time, fed up with it all. The medical appointments were relentless, and the toll of chemotherapy was starting to show. I was tired, I was emotional, and my tolerance levels had fallen drastically. I was pretty much rushed from one treatment to another. I had barely a three week break from finishing chemo to starting radiation. In hindsight, I should have given myself more time, but I was like 'no time like the present'. I just wanted to get it over with.

There was nothing that could have prepared me for that part of the ongoing treatment for cancer. It didn't matter what anyone said to me, the fear had risen up to the point I was frozen in my own body. I suffered agonising panic attacks during treatment, I was a mess.

Barely one person in that department cared enough to see that I was slowly unravelling; I was just another patient, just another person coming in and out every day. Another faceless person. It was so awful I became physically sick just turning round the street corner on my way to the hospital. I was like Pavlov's dog in reverse, as soon as I saw the building the nausea would rise up and I would look for the closest bin to vomit in.

The staff huddled in their little rooms, out of sight of the patients. The corridors were empty, it was eerie. At the time of day I went there, the cleaners were about the only people I saw, wheeling their bins around silently like a horror movie. To make matters worse, I had to parade around the corridors and hallways in a dressing gown. How hideous and undignified, it was worse than wearing a prison uniform. I hated the fact I had to undress every time I went for treatment, I hated being naked in that horrible room full of gigantic machines. I was so embarrassed.

I know the people working there had seen it all before, but I hadn't. I wasn't used to this amount of exposure. Why couldn't I have been covered up? You cannot tell me that radiation can't get through a piece of fabric? Why do I have to be naked? This was never explained to me, you just had to do what they told you. It added to my anxiety every day I went.

Every session was the same, I would be shuffled around the table for ten minutes, people touching me and my breasts all the time. I really hated it. I refused the tattoos—that was a given—I was not going to be pressured into getting permanent skin markings for treatment. There was no way I wanted a permanent reminder of radiation; it had been said that, "Radiation tattoos are your mark of survival." You have to be joking. Who wants a reminder of being a breast cancer patient?

I felt invisible. My concerns went unanswered, there was no information about how to cope with the horrendous treatment, and they gave me no information about how to look after my skin, which by the start of week three had macerated and was extremely painful. I couldn't sleep, I couldn't eat, I was in a constant state of anxiety. It had risen up and was holding me hostage.

I endured sixteen sessions of hypo-fractioned radiotherapy and on the last day of treatment I cried because I was so sad, so angry, so hopeless, and in a lot of pain. The kind of pain I had never experienced before. I couldn't get out of there quick enough, I was panic-stricken.

I sat in the park after my last treatment and cried until the sun started to fall beyond the horizon.

The park had beautiful daffodils all poking their heads up and waving in the wind. I felt like a child again, sitting on the bench curled up watching the flowers; I used to love doing that, it brought me comfort. It was starting to get cold but I couldn't move from the park bench. I was petrified. I rugged up in my coat and hat and buried my head in my hood. How did this happen?

I felt worse now than I ever had. I was exhausted, my poor body was wilting. I had so far been cut opened, systematically poisoned, and now my skin was so burnt I could feel the heat radiating out of my chest like I was on fire. My skin was burning from the inside out, and I thought I was going to pass out from the pain.

I stayed on that park bench for an hour, by that time it was dark and cold. I had to go home, it was over, I never had to go back there again. That was the only reason I hauled myself off that bench. It was over. No more of those people, no more of that awful place again, ever. I swore that day I would never put myself through radiotherapy again.

But I did have to pick myself up and get serious about finding help for the inner torment and panic attacks.

Before I could attempt anything 'mindful' I had to treat the physical side effects; my skin was peeling off and red raw, I needed medical attention. My safe space was at my GP's rooms, I couldn't return to the hospital—that was out of the question. Without a doubt, the resident nurse at my GP's surgery is an angel; she helped me at a time of real need. It was so comforting to see a familiar face, a face I had seen on the very day I was diagnosed. A person who really cared about me, who wanted to help me, who knew my family and my children, someone who knew what to do.

I was given 'burn victim' gel to lather myself in, and it was instant relief from the heat. I was so grateful that day. Grateful I had finished radiation but even more grateful someone had showed me so much kindness. I was overwhelmed by the care I received, she was a shining light in a place that had gotten awfully dark.

One week after I finished the last session of radiation the pain was continuing to be so excruciating that I thought something had gone horribly wrong. My skin was even redder than the week before, and skin was peeling off underneath my breast. My armpit was so painful I now couldn't put my arm down by my side. I could barely move it. Everything I wore rubbed on my skin and even the unflattering soft fabric crop tops were too painful to even attempt to put on. How was I going to go to work and do my normal things with no bra on? Impossible. My breasts would be hanging down near my belly button if I did, and I would be so embarrassed to go out in public bra-less.

I ended up making a sort of sling from an old t-shirt that supported me, but kept the skin from smarting and rubbing. I felt like someone from the 1800s, before bras were invented. I can't believe it was the year 2016 and there was nothing out there I could buy that would support my breast and cool the searing heat it was radiating.

I seriously thought of using those things you put in your lunch box to keep your food cold; those frozen floppy gel packs. At least they were cold, maybe I could put one inside the make shift bra?

The only problem was they leaked water as they were melting and would make my top wet after a while. Back to the drawing board—I was prepared to try anything! If I could have put my breast in the freezer I would have.

I found out later the worst time for radiation is one week after, then it supposedly starts to settle down.

Wow! No one at the hospital told me my skin would be totally barbecued after the last session of radiation, and even worse a week later. If I had known then I would have been prepared for it, at least I would have known what was coming.

I don't know how many times before my treatment I told the specialist at the hospital I was concerned about my skin. I have very pale skin, and I was very worried about skin damage. I am the type of person who goes out in summer with a long sleeve top and a hat. My skin cannot tolerate even ten minutes in the sun. And here I was subjecting myself to external beam radiation.

"Oh, it's just like a bit of sunburn," the specialist said.

No. It's not like a bit of sunburn, it's like a second-degree burn. Big difference. I wondered how he would cope with second-degree burns on his penis.

Even having a shower was painful; if the water even slightly sprayed on my skin, it would feel like little bullets being fired at me. I would be doing a little hopping dance, flapping my arms around, while waiting for the pain to subside. I had to cup the water spray with my other hand and gently try to wash the left side of me.

I took so much care not to bump my left side; even the slightest brush past a fellow commuter would send pain radiating through my skin. I had to re-evaluate my travelling plans on the train during that time, I stopped getting the crowded express trains because I couldn't take the risk of someone accidentally bumping into me. It wouldn't have been their fault, but I had to take action to protect myself and that meant taking the slow train home from work every day and adding an hour to my trip. It made for a long working week when my poor body was trying desperately to heal itself.

I chose to work full time the whole way through radiation, a choice I do not regret. While I may have been in pain physically, not working and lying on the sofa at home thinking about what had happened to me those past few weeks was worse for my mental health. I was determined to have a reason to get up in the morning, and determined I wasn't going to let this stop my life.

I would make my radiation sessions at the end of the day, usually 5pm, so I could work all day, then go there after work, and then go straight home. It kept my mind busy to be at work and gave me the opportunity to do normal things and not talk about cancer. I welcomed the normalcy. Only a few people at work knew about my cancer diagnosis, so it was important for me to be seen as doing all the normal things I would. Saying that, it was becoming very draining towards the end. I was fatigued from the treatment and my anxiety had risen to stratospheric levels, keeping it together became quite difficult.

I woke up every morning dreading the end of the day when I would have to go back to the torture chamber. I seriously thought of never going back, that thought had crossed my mind many, many times. I was told if I didn't finish the course of treatment it wouldn't work. It's not like you can do half and get half the benefit. You have to do the whole course. I was over half way through and I had already endured ten treatments so that would have all been in vain if I gave up then.

Talk about not having an option. I had to get through the rest of the treatment, otherwise I would not have completed it all and would not get the benefit of killing off any stray cancer cells. What a desperately awful situation. I had no choice but to continue.

I willed time to go quickly, just another week and I would be OK. It was the longest week of my life. There is nothing in this world that could make me have radiation treatment again, it is barbaric, and I will never subject myself to it again, full stop.

It was around then I really thought about all the people I had encountered along the way, and there were so many of them. Overwhelming, in fact, just how many people are involved in your cancer care. It's called your 'treatment team'.

I would be much more receptive to this term if it meant my 'beauty treatment team', which included a manicure, pedicure, and facial. I was not interested in having a medical oncologist, radiation oncologist, an occupational therapist, a dietician, radiation therapist, etc. The list goes on, and on.

Too many. It was mind boggling and I struggled with not only the frequency of appointments to see all those people, but the standard of care was vastly different between each specialist, nurse, doctor, etc. In total I had already seen sixteen different specialists, sixteen! And that didn't include all the nursing staff who had assisted me through chemotherapy. I actually had never heard of half of these specialists, why would I? Whoever thinks they are going to need a radiation oncologist or a lymphedema therapist? No one.

Just the sheer logistics of making an appointment with those people was exhausting enough on top of your treatment and generally trying to deal with a cancer diagnosis. Then, trying to fit the appointments into a full time work schedule was almost impossible.

I would frequently receive phone calls from the specialist's rooms, along the lines of, "We have booked you in to see the doctor at quarter past two."

"Ahh, no, I work full time," I said. "Unless you can fit me in at eight am or five pm, then I can't come."

That was a regular conversation, one I had many times. It was almost impossible to fit appointments in around working. I would often have an appointment at 5pm, which was great, but it still meant I had to leave work at 4pm—an hour before I was supposed to finish, and an hour more personal leave to take.

On a good week, I would have maybe two appointments, but some weeks I could realistically have four.

My week would go like this: Monday 5pm, oncologist. Tuesday 9am, radiation oncologist. Thursday 8am, blood tests. Friday 10.30am, oncology ward for treatment.

All of that while managing a team of people, as well as a department assisting the business, which turned over millions of dollars.

While some specialists were very accommodating with my appointments, some didn't budge. And the ones who didn't budge couldn't even keep their appointment time. The 9.30am could well turn into a 10.15am, making me three hours late for work. Another three hours of personal leave, another several hundred dollars out of my bank account, another inflexible specialist and—oops! Aren't I the patient?

Sometimes things just have to be said. I was tested to the max with constant concerns and constant pressures to be at one appointment or another, one treatment or another, and I think it is really OK to have a moment of insanity. It would have been weird if I didn't.

It was such a stressful time; you need stamina, you need grace, you need understanding. I forget sometimes about the enormity of what I have already been through. I'm awesome to have gone through it; it would just be nice sometimes if medical specialists said it to me too.

I don't want to seem ungrateful. I am grateful for their expertise, and their years of study, and that the treatment they prescribed for me is possibly saving my life, but I feel some of them have 'compassion fatigue'.

I totally understand caring for people with cancer must be draining and cause emotional stress—I couldn't do that job, I know I wouldn't be up to the challenge. But if you choose that profession, then I think it is very important that caring for others is on the top of your list, your top priority. Because as a cancer patient, I know when someone doesn't give a shit. It is obvious. There is a very noticeable difference between the angels and the, 'I don't give a shit' person. Actually it's a very wide chasm.

The downside to being on Herceptin is the three monthly heart tests (along with your treatment being nine months longer). Herceptin can increase your risk of congestive heart failure and decrease how well the heart pumps blood out of its main pumping chamber, the left ventricle. I know, another side effect! Another way that cancer keeps on giving.

So that meant regular echo-cardiograms. More appointments, more people to see, more money flowing out of my account, and more awkward and embarrassing tests. I had six echo-cardiograms in total, but my experience with those tests was different.

The only reason was because the person who did the echo tests for me was beautiful in every sense of the word. She was not only calm, compassionate and tranquil; she was so peaceful in her demeanour. I had never met anyone at the radiology department who showed that amount of care, I was shocked. I had prepared myself for the worst, quite frankly; I had some pretty harrowing experiences. She was so interested in me, in just me. She was a great listener, asked relevant questions about how I was feeling, seemed genuinely interested in how I was coping with the treatment, and told me stories of other breast cancer survivors. Whether she meant it or not, she told me all the good stories, only positivity.

I wanted to tell her everything... everything on my mind; she was the first person who had been receptive to my questions and feedback. I told her all about the dreadful service I received at the radiology department and she was shocked. She said it wasn't right—indeed it wasn't, but it had happened. I could tell she was a spiritual person, and a book worm, just like me.

While I was waiting for my next round of tests she came back to me and handed me a piece of paper. It was a list of books; on the bottom of the note was a drawing of a heart, just like the heart chakra, the heart centre. She had given me love, given me a strong heart through her own compassion. She said that you can always choose love, and she was right.

When you feel fear, you cannot feel love, and vice versa. I had the power inside me to change my feelings, to change my perception. What a beautiful person. I will never forget her; an angel walked into my life and left a trail, a trail of enlightenment to what I truly could do to heal myself, and my mind.

I wrote an email to the radiology centre, giving them feedback on my experiences; I singled out the one person who had been of the utmost comfort at a very distressing time, but also told them about the many failings of the rest of their services and people they employ. I never got a response back.

It was the second time I had given feedback, and the first time I didn't get a response, either. Why do these establishments ask for feedback? Do they only want good feedback? What is the point of giving feedback, if they only use it to tell the public about the high percentage of satisfied customers?

I provided my name and contact details on both feedback surveys, I wasn't anonymous. I wanted them to contact me, I wanted them to ask me why my experience had been poor. They were not interested.

I am still available if they want to contact me.

# CHAPTER 21

When I started practicing yoga regularly, I saw the indigo chakra, the third eye chakra. It was vivid and beautiful in my mind, and it was perfect. I know it sounds a bit 'new age' and something I would probably have pooh-poohed myself previously, but it was an amazing experience. I cannot put into words how it made me feel, it was like nothing I had experienced before. Similar to a sixth sense, I was mesmerised by the visions. I had never seen such an exquisite colour.

I knew it had to mean something, how could the vision not be a sign of my senses awaking and realising a deeper existence? The last six months of my life had truly been a roller-coaster of terrifying emotions. I was so disconnected with myself; I didn't even really know who I was. I had no clarity, no insight, and I couldn't see the big picture of my life. I was shattered and anxious. My life was falling apart.

Chakras by definition are energy centres within the human body that help to regulate all of its processes, from the immune system, to organ function and emotions.

Originating from Sanskrit, it means 'wheel' and spinning energy. It all meant very little to me, modern medicine does not support the existence of chakras, let alone what they are capable of doing. Eastern medicine is not new, in fact it is very old, older than western medicine. Eastern nations all over the world practice the energy flow and know exactly how they can benefit the human body. A negative outlook on life obstructs the 'spin' of those wheels and that results in sickness, illness, and disease.

The great majority of health issues today are created in the mental and emotional state. We live lives that are stressed, forever hectic, and we suppress emotional hurting. We hold onto the past, we lie, we are jealous; we turn things over and over in our minds until we make ourselves sick. We are burnt-out, exhausted, and fearful. Our energy stops flowing and gets stuck in our body. If not dealt with, then we destroy and deplete our body of life energy.

My life energy was definitely stuck, I just didn't know it.

Cancer struck me, and it affected every area of my life, physically, emotionally, psychologically, and spiritually.

It has been said that indigo-coloured energy is the energy of deep change—so as you unfold the petals of the third eye chakra, you begin to recognise patterns; you can see where you have been, where you are stuck and where you are going.

Tears flowed out of the corners of my eyes when I saw the beautiful vision. I realised I was experiencing a sense of tranquilly and completeness, it was life changing.

The Indigo Chakra is symbolised by the lotus flower, as all chakras are, each with a different number of petals. The Indigo Chakra flower has two petals; I now call them the 'old me' and the 'new me'.

It was time for Ruby's books again. I loved Ruby, she is immensely funny and I could really relate to her and her humour. I had never been a particular fan of 'self-help' books, I knew the titles of some of the more well-known authors, but at that time I didn't need to read books about earning more money, or getting more customers, or finding religion. I needed help from someone who knew what it was like to fall into the hurricane of depression, someone who knew what it was like to be depleted and broken.

I obviously don't know Ruby personally but I have learnt a lot about her through her books, and a lot of what she said resonated with me. Her chapter on 'critical voices' is really thought provoking. So why are we so mean to ourselves? She talks about how we are so hard on ourselves, we are in fact our own worst enemies.

I was guilty of that ten times over. I constantly beat myself up, it was never ending and it was playing over in my mind like a broken record. I was attacking myself every day, hurting myself every day—no wonder mental illness is on the rise. That is a scary notion and one that I had thought about a lot.

I would honestly have days when it was all I thought about, negative thoughts would swirl in my head constantly. I would replay events that happened over and over trying to think of ways I could do things better. What I would say to people who had wronged me, people who didn't care—it was exhausting and I didn't know how to stop the toxic thoughts. Even yoga at the moment wasn't helping. Nothing was, and I was terrified I had finally lost it.

Finding solace in books was just what I needed. It was familiar; it was my way of switching off from the world just as I had done many times before. Losing myself in another world, the world of imagination. I did it as a child, a teenager, a young adult; books were always there, like a friend I could call on at any time of the day or night. A constant companion.

I didn't want to talk to people about how I was feeling. I didn't want to see a psychologist; I wanted to understand it myself. I wanted to know how I could make my brain better myself, I knew I had it in me. I might have been spiritually and mentally broken, anxious and barely holding it together, but I knew deep down inside that I had the tools to do it, I just needed to know how.

From Ruby's book I realised I needed to practice noticing things around me more and make it a habit. Wow, OK, now that was a revelation to me, the mindfulness stuff continues to be a theme running through a lot of books I've read. I know this sounds all a bit mumbo jumbo but I was desperate to learn about how to calm my mind. There had to be a way, there had to be an instructional manual, a step by step guide on how to stop the worry, stop the fear, stop the shame. Stop all those negative-Nancy voices swirling around in my head.

# CHAPTER 22

My dear (and until recently, absent) friend sensed I needed some help. I don't know how but she knew I wasn't in the right 'head space', maybe it was the crazy lady way I was talking, maybe it was the constant jabbering, I subjected her to about everything and anything.

She knew exactly what to say to me. She had been there, the confusing world of not knowing where you are heading, having no direction, coasting along on automatic pilot.

She said I needed to focus—to focus on personal development and growing my mind. I had visions of planted watermelon seeds in my brain and watching the vines grow out my ears. What exactly is growing your mind?

Thankfully, what was growing was the hair on my body. Tiny little hairs were popping up almost overnight. My eyelashes and eyebrows were finally starting to look 'normal' (whatever that is!) again. I had stopped going to the eyebrow parlour because on the last visit when she went to give me a head massage, little eyebrow hairs were lifting and sticking to her fingers—how embarrassing.

I said it was the menopause, I didn't want to have the whole conversation with someone I barely knew and it was an open salon, so everyone could have heard me.

For the past six months I had practically drawn on my eyebrows every morning. I can tell you at 6.30am on a cold winter morning, attempting to draw on perfect eyebrows was impossible. I was no good at it. My daughters watch YouTube videos of people doing their eyebrows so they can nail it perfectly; I needed to do some of my own studying on the technique. I never ever thought I would have to be perfecting eyebrow drawing, not once. I usually left them right alone. I knew too many friends who had over plucked them in their teenage years and they never grew back properly.

My eyelashes didn't completely fall out, just little chunks, so they could be covered with a bit of skilled mascara application. I was however, disappointed when the hairs on my legs started growing back. Bummer, it was one of the only good side effects.

As summer approached, the hot flushes were getting unbearable. I started calling them my 'sweaty Betty's'. I took to buying extra paper fans and distributing them everywhere that I went; the car, the lounge room, the family room, bedside table, desk at work, and my handbag. I couldn't be without the $2.00 miracle worker. It became a bit of a joke at work when I madly flipped out my paper fan to cool myself down in a meeting.

"It's just the menopause," I would say. Five minutes later and I was fine, it was the most bizarre thing. It would start in my face first. I would go all red from the neck up and then start sweating around my hairline, and finally down my spine. I felt so overcome with heat sometimes, I thought I would pass out. Totally embarrassing when you are trying to conduct a staff review.

I suffered mostly at night time, which hugely disrupted my sleep. I would wake at least four times a night covered in sweat. I would flip the doona off and starfish in bed. Five minutes later, and I was shivering from my sweat going cold so the doona ended up back around my ears.

It continued for months and months until I was absolutely

exhausted form lack of restful sleep. Yoga was supposed to help, and maybe it had, I could have been getting it ten times worse. Who knows?

I got to a point one hot humid night where I just sat on the floor and cried. I was so hot, so tired, and hated everything about menopause, it wasn't fair. I had been hit so hard with the effects of chemotherapy killing off my ovaries that the symptoms seemed to be tenfold.

I wasn't coping with this disruption to my life every hour on the hour, seven days a week. It was relentless and the hot flushes were starting to be preceded by nausea too. It was getting worse. I guess the only good thing was at least I got an early warning the hot flush was coming. The wave of nausea would last about twenty seconds and then one minute later I would start sweating.

Day in day out, it was the same; I found it extremely hard to do normal things like cooking. The heat from the gas top or stove would exacerbate the heat coming out of my face. How much more could I take?

The last few months were taking their toll; nausea, fatigue, bloody noses, weak and broken nails, diarrhoea, burnt skin, disappearing veins, brittle hair, spotty skin, and dizziness. Was there anything else that could be thrown at me? My poor body was broken and now it was leaking water all the time.

I knew very little about the 'change in life'. I hadn't banked on going through menopause for at least a few more years. I was blissfully unaware at how debilitating it could be. Some literature I read said that many women believe menopause is not only a physical transformation, but a spiritual and emotional one in which you emerge wiser and more intuitive. Bullshit. I was soaked in my own sweat and cranky as all hell, I did not feel like I was entering the 'wise women' years. Far from it.

I asked my specialist what I could take for the menopause; the answer was pretty much nothing, No Hormone Replacement Therapy (HRT) for me. Oh, but I could take some low dose antidepressants. They may help, but it would take a few months to kick in, and I could not just stop taking them. You need to be weaned off them. In addition, it had been documented that antidepressants have side effects also, which include agitation, diarrhoea, insomnia, and bone loss. They seemed worse than the hot flushes I was trying to get rid of. Antidepressants didn't seem like a very good choice to me. Taking more pills, no thanks, I was already taking Tamoxifen daily; I really didn't want to be relying on more pills with more possible side effects.

But I was desperate, I needed something to tame those hot flushes, they were debilitating by that stage and the summer weather wasn't helping at all. My specialist did say that I could try acupuncture.

"There have been some good results from acupuncture and the symptoms of menopause," she said. "You could always give it a try."

I would have given anything at that stage a try quite frankly; if they had told me sitting backwards on a horse and riding around in circles would work, I would have tried it.

I remember my yoga teacher telling me about a Chinese medicine doctor who did acupuncture so I decided to ask her about him. She spoke of him regularly and how he had helped people she knew overcome all sorts of things. Vertigo, infertility, soft tissue injury, etc. and she believed he could solve my menopause problems.

I must say I was a bit dubious about it all. I had been to an acupuncturist before to try and stop smoking, and while I do remember feeling a sense of well-being after the treatments I didn't continue because it wasn't working on my addiction. I was still smoking ten a day and had no feeling of wanting to stop. Plus, I remember the foul tasting tea she gave me and that wasn't something I was happy to revisit.

So, with trepidation, I made an appointment to see the Chinese medicine doctor. His brochure did say that he treats, "Abnormality of internal organs according to TCM; menopausal syndrome." Well, I had absolutely nothing to lose.

My first appointment was quite long, which was to be expected. He didn't know me, and we had to chat about all things from my cancer diagnosis, previous surgeries, energy levels, sleep patterns, etc. and then he spoke to me about Yin and Yang which I totally didn't understand. Apparently my kidneys were unbalanced and I need to get my yin and yang back to where it should be. I had no idea what that meant.

He stuck four acupuncture needles in my stomach and one in particular was really quite painful. I don't know exactly which meridian it was poked into but geez it hurt. He said to relax for twenty minutes, which was hard to do when there were four needles poking out of my stomach, one of which felt like it had been drilled down into my kidney.

After the twenty minutes had passed he came back and took the needles out before giving me a small container of powder. Oh, yuck, it was that horrible tea again. The label said it had six ingredients, which meant nothing to me. Just lots of botanical names and a bitter smell.

"Take three spoons, three times a day before meals and come back and see me next week."

OK, so I had a few needles stuck in me and then had to drink the smelly brew for a week—was that it? Well, I thought I better look into it a bit more so I could understand what the heck all this Traditional Chinese Medicine was about.

Traditional Chinese Medicine (TCM) is vastly different from western medicine; firstly it treats the person as a whole, not just one part of you.

Traditional Chinese medicine is based on the theory that all of the body's organs mutually support each other. Therefore, in order to be healthy, an individual's organs, and their functions must be in balance. This balance is attained, in part, by harmonizing yin and yang, two opposing but complementary energies thought to affect all life.

Another theory in traditional Chinese medicine is that vital energy (called "qi" or "chi") flows throughout the body via certain pathways (or "meridians"). According to this theory, disease and other emotional, mental, and physical health problems develop when the flow of qi is blocked, weak, or excessive. Restoring the flow of qi is considered essential to balancing the yin and yang and, in turn, achieving wellness.

OK, it was all quite interesting. I never really had any interest in eastern medicine, I only fleetingly knew some principles but nothing much more than that. I was intrigued about the flow of energy. Yoga had opened my mind to the possibility of the invisible energy laneways. I certainly felt a lot better, whether it was through my treatment, or afterwards while I was recovering. I had started feeling a certain wellness I couldn't really put my finger on.

Maybe it was my meridians? In India, the yogis call energy, prana, and the energy pathways, nadis. In china it is called qi, and the pathways are called meridians, which is what founded the science of acupuncture. So it is kind of the same thing, yoga and acupuncture. Both are unblocking the highways of energy flowing through the body. Of course you can't see the pathways, which could be why western medicine has been rather sceptical of it all; there is no physical evidence of it.

I mainly practice Yin Yoga, I find that type of yoga the most beneficial for me because it is a passive practice that involves variations of poses either seated, or on your back, which you typically hold for three to five minutes. It's better for a beginner because it gives you the chance to slow down and isn't too taxing on the body. Once you are in the pose, you can relax and breathe into yourself and just 'be'. I loved it a lot when I first started and I love it even more now. There is a certain feeling of serenity and peace in the very calming practice. Our teacher talks about the three Yin Yoga tenants:

1. Find a suitable edge, as you enter your pose, move slowly and gently into the shape. Pause and listen to your body.

2. Be still, don't fix or change your pose. Resolve not to fidget.

3. Hold for a while, hold your pose for three to five minutes. You don't need comfort to feel at ease, instead of contracting around feelings and sensation, just breathe.

Yin Yoga stretches your connective tissue, although that might sound painful it's not. It's not about straining anything or bending the wrong way, you work with your body to promote flexibility in the main areas of your body like your hips, pelvis, and lower spine. Yin Yoga is not strenuous exercise, it is calming and meditative, and it was the best 'find' of my life.

Between yoga and acupuncture I cannot tell you how fantastic I started feeling. By the time I had been practicing yoga for six months, not only was I getting good at those pretzel poses, I was noticeably feeling the benefits.

Chinese medical practitioners and yogis have insisted that blocks to the flow of vital energy throughout our body eventually manifest in physical problems that would seem, on the surface, to have nothing to do with weak knees or a stiff back. There needs to be more research conducted to confirm the relationship between yoga and TCM, but if yoga postures really do help us reach down into the body and gently stimulate the flow of qi and prana through the connective tissue, Yin Yoga serves as a tool for helping you get the greatest possible benefit from yoga practice.

Coping with the sweaty Betty's was still a huge problem, even in yoga classes. Trying to wipe my brow of sweat while being in a downward facing dog was extremely hard, I just ended up dripping sweat pools on the yoga mat. Luckily, I had been given a yoga mat for Mother's Day; at least I wasn't dripping sweat on someone else's mat.

The first time I took the 'menopause tea' (which is what I called it) I nearly gagged. It was disgusting. It was so bitter it took my breath away. I had to have a fruit juice 'chaser' after I drank it so the taste would move out of my mouth. I screwed my face up like a child given a Brussel sprout to eat. This stuff was so gross I could hardly get it near my mouth before my gag reflex would start, and I had to do it three times a day for three months. I could barely get it down for three seconds.

My Chinese doctor said, "Just wait and see, you'll see."

But see what, exactly? I was curious, but also slightly sceptical about all of it. Time would tell, I just had to get that damn tea down my throat.

As far as Chinese medicine views menopause, it couldn't be more different than western medicine. Treating problems associated with menopause through Chinese medicine involves tonifying and balancing the kidney function with acupuncture and/or Chinese herbal medicine. When Kidney Yin is deficient the body will lack fluid, or will become dry and will easily overheat. Therefore, Chinese herbs that nourish and clear the heat are given. When Kidney Yang is deficient there is not enough warmth and too much fluid in the body. Therefore, Yang tonifying and warming herbs are prescribed.

I remember my yoga teacher talking about Yin and Yang, the

symbol for it has two equal parts, one black and one white. The black is yang and the yin, white, but each has a tiny circle of the opposing colour in each, like a pair of eyes. Apparently there is always a little bit of yin in the yang and vice versa.

I could certainly relate to that when I was doing Yin Yoga, because when I had been in a pose for five minutes, and my hamstrings were screaming at me, that was my little bit of yang.

The circles of Yin and Yang are also symbols of cycles that represent the old saying of what comes around goes around. Literature tells us as humans, we have the capacity for greatness but also for great destruction. I guess that is what makes us stand on the line of being only just in control sometimes.

The goal of life is to hold it together, at any time we can trip up, tip over the edge. I certainly had been there many times over the past twelve months. I had seen myself as many things; sometimes I was whole, sometimes I moved between the light and the dark, a bit like the white and black of Yin and Yang.

I got it. It's OK, to swing between those two shades of life, its actually OK to have those thoughts. We all have them, it's in our nature, I just had to acknowledge the thoughts that arose and choose whether I held on to them. "Don't try too hard, trying is an effort, it's natural, just like sleep is natural." Be kind to yourself.

It was a whole new world for me but I could see the juxtaposition, the connection to this practice, Yin and Yang, a positive force and a negative force working in harmony with each other. Light and dark, I had my fair share of both.

It was draining and when I felt another hot flush coming I started getting anxious again, especially if I was on a crowded train on my way home. All that talk about kidney heat had to mean something. Were my kidneys hot? Was that what was making me sweaty? Goodness knows, but if my yin and yang are out then that could be the reason?

I'm not sure how you know your yin and yang are not aligned; I guess that is what the Chinese doctor does. It's invisible, but I understand it can cause imbalance; I certainly had way too much heat happening in my body. I could have saved on the electricity bill and heated the house just by the sheer heat radiating out of my body. Given, I still had a barbecued boob from the radiation treatment.

I was emitting so much heat out of every surface of my body, I should have changed my name to Blaze.

## CHAPTER 23

My scepticism of this Chinese medicine stuff lasted for the first few months, I felt no different. I was pouring the gross tea down my throat three times a day and having acupuncture every second week. The sense of well-being continued but the sweaty Betty's were still coming thick and fast. I had resigned myself to the fact that I was going to have to live with it, regardless.

I didn't know if my menopause was caused by taking the Tamoxifen, or by my shrivelled ovaries, but whatever was causing it was still there and I really had just about given up. The regular visits to the Chinese doctor were becoming tiresome as he was not close to my home or work, and I had spent quite a lot of money. I was just about to call and cancel my next appointment.

I cannot put it down to a particular day but one morning I got out of bed and realised I had not woken up during the night profusely sweating. In fact, I had not woken up at all.

Wow, I mean wow! I had not done that in nine months. What a miracle. I was worried it might have just been a 'one hit wonder' so I was looking forward to going to bed again the next night to see what happened.

Again, I slept right through.

I tracked myself for a week, no sweating during the night. Whatever was in the tea was working; my overheated kidneys were cooling down. I started to feel human again. I was still having hot flushes during the day, but it was less and less frequent. Hours would go past and I would think, "I haven't had a hot flush!" I could sit in a meeting and not be rummaging around for a fan. I wasn't stripping all my clothes off on the train.

It was very gradual, but after six months of taking the tea and other special formulas of Chinese herb stems and leaves, the sweaty Betty's had subsided by at least 90%. My Chinese medicine doctor is a wizard. It was magic.

I would not have believed it if someone had told me in six months the menopause symptoms would be almost gone. I was in awe of how it really worked; an ancient practice had helped me enormously in the 21st century. I don't have to take the tea anymore, just a few capsules a day to keep my yin and yang balanced, but I will be forever grateful for whatever was in that witches brew.

And I am not sure I ever want to know.

I was amassing a pile of self-help books of all denominations, and was enjoying reading them. They were uplifting and much better than reading scary cancer stories on the Internet.

Sometimes I found myself slipping back into familiar territory, I would Google, 'breast cancer', and see what popped up but nine out of ten times it was something depressing. I had to stop, it wasn't helping.

I would find myself typing 'reoccurrence', 'HER2, 'cancer prognosis', it was a bit obsessive really. I realised that there was a lesson right here for me, and whatever I needed would be revealed to me, I had to trust myself, not Dr. Google.

I decided it was like reading the newspaper, there was only going to be bad stories. I vowed I would stop again. If my mind was full of all these negative things, how was I going to say positive? You cannot have both of those feelings at the same time. It's impossible.

I chose to be positive and try at least ninety percent of the time to think happy things. That didn't mean that I didn't have crap days when I was back to Googling scary cancer stories, but my mindset was changing. I felt so much better when I read something positive and uplifting and the exact opposite when I read something negative. You don't have to be a rocket scientist to work that one out, you feel good when you are happy.

I happened across a book called *The Power of Now* by Eckhart Tolle. The book had been recommended to me twice. Once, by my serene yoga teacher, and once, from the angel who did my echocardiograms. After two people had mentioned the book to me, I thought I had better have a look at it. I had never heard of it but apparently it is a best seller and Tolle is known as a contemporary spiritual teacher.

Tolle tells of how the book has transformed people's lives. He receives letters from people all over the world telling him how they have found tranquillity and inner peace. I was keen to see what he had to say. Hold onto that thought. I finished reading it, and didn't understand a word of it, so I am on my second round of reading.

We rush through our lives every day and never stop to take in what is happening around us. I had finally finished reading the *Power of Now* (for the third time) and read that in 2011 Eckhart Tolle was listed as "the most spiritually influential person in the world." Interestingly, it is not an easy book to read. I found the concepts hard to understand, but realise now that our brains are just not wired that way and we learn that behaviour from a very young age.

The main message of the book, as I see it was to realise that the present moment is all we ever have. I really had to think about that. You only have now, your past was a now, your future is a now, it's all a now. Recognising how you feel right here and now is quite the strangest thing, you concentrate on what you are actually feeling or doing at that moment. It is calming, it has no memory attached to it, and it just is. There is a great comfort in the realization; enjoy what you have right now, it is perfect.

The primary cause of unhappiness is never the situation but the thought about it. Apparently we need to separate our thoughts from what is happening around us, we are only ever right here, right now. I needed to be aware of the thoughts I was thinking so in my head I could separate the two. Training my brain to not project my past thoughts and experiences into the future is difficult, it has taken me quite some time to get my head around the concept.

While I had been lucky with the scalp cooling, my hair had become quite dry and brittle by the end of chemotherapy, so I just left it for a while. But it really needed cutting. I booked in with my hairdresser and said, "I need something different, something fabulous!" And that was what she did.

My hair had been halfway down my back during treatment, and she cut it back to my shoulders. I was very happy, I sort of looked like a new me with shorter hair. It felt great to have a haircut after months of treating my hair with kid gloves. I have been a redhead all my life, and I am very proud of my mutation.

Redheads make up only 1-2% of the world's population, and my combination of red hair and green eyes is even rarer. Saving my hair was so important to me; my hair had always been my crowning glory. It was a mixture of gold and red and it was slightly wavy. My hair was me. I get that some people think, 'it is only hair, it will grow back', but unless you are faced with the real possibility your hair might fall out, you cannot have an opinion. Unless you know what it is like to lose your identity (regardless of what you think about hair and identity), losing your hair is traumatic.

As the months went on after finishing chemo, the hair that had fallen out started to sprout. The funniest thing for me was that because I hadn't lost all of my hair, the new hair was growing in between the old hair. Now that might not seem strange except for the fact that the new hair was growing back a different colour. I had read that hair grows back in all different guises after chemotherapy, mostly that it grows back curly or grey! Mine grew back blonde. Nothing like my natural colour at all.

I am not sure what I was expecting really, but I didn't think it would grow back a totally different colour. I now have blonde highlights (for want of a better word); twenty percent of my hair looked like I had professional foils done, bonus!

# CHAPTER 24

In Jennifer Saunders' book *Bonkers* she mentions that after her cancer treatment she got a dog. She talks about how it was great therapy for what she had been through, and I hadn't forgotten reading about how her dog had come into her life.

I had grown up with dogs, my mum picked up any stray animal roaming the streets when we were children. Our house was like a menagerie; at one point we had four cats and fours dogs at home, more animals than children.

I had longed for a dog for quite a while but work commitments prevented us from getting one as no one was home during the day. I was walking a lot more these days, just getting out in nature buoyed my mood and stopped me from churning thoughts of cancer over and over in my head. It was therapeutic to be out pounding the pavement, but I felt like I was missing something.

It hit me. I needed a dog. A dog to walk with, a dog to care for and love, a furry friend to need me. I too, wanted the same experience as Jennifer.

My husband knew I wanted a dog, and what a surprise that he presented me with a 'one small dog' voucher for my forty-eighth birthday. I cried, I was so grateful. That was all I wanted for my birthday, the birthday I turned forty-eight and left forty-seven (the age when I was diagnosed) behind. It was a milestone for me to turn forty-eight, and with the year of my birthday changing over, I felt released from that time in my life. And now I had the chance to own a dog.

Raffy could not have been more perfect. He was just how I imagined him; small, white, and scruffy. I knew I would always have a rescue dog, my parents had instilled in us there are too many abandoned dogs that need a good home, so it was right for me to head to the Lost Dogs Home to find my perfect pooch.

My oldest daughter and I headed out of town one Saturday morning to meet potential furry family members. The dog we arranged to see from the Internet photo was not suitable. I was disappointed because I had in my mind I would take a dog home that day and I thought he would be perfect. But just as we were leaving I spied a small white dog in the corner enclosure that was out of bounds for visitors.

I enquired about the two dogs who were peering out from behind the cage and was told they had just arrived and hadn't been checked over by the vet, so they were in isolation for a week until that had happened. They weren't up for adoption.

I could see this small, white scruffy dog just like in my imagination. He was perfect. I asked if I could see him and they obliged, but said that he had an eye problem and they weren't sure if he was partially blind or whether his weeping eyes would be an ongoing problem that would need daily treatment. I didn't care; he was exactly the dog for me.

As soon as they let him out for me to meet I knew that he would be part of our family. They didn't know what type of dog he was, a mutt, bits and pieces of all breeds. He had very small legs like a corgi, white fluffy fur like a Pomeranian, and a pointy face like a Jack Russell; he was indeed a blend of many breeds. He was smiling when he met my daughter and I; the grin on his face expressed his inner dog thoughts. I wanted to take him home straight away, but I had to wait until he had been cleared. In the meantime, I was told if someone else came out to the lost dog's home once he had been checked over, he could be adopted by someone else!

I called every day to see when he would be ready, and one week later, on the eve of Halloween, I got to take him home. He's perfect in every way, though he does have weepy eyes, which leave stains on his fur where his eyes continually run. But he is the most cheerful little dog, and I love having him in my life. I now have a walking partner and I couldn't be happier.

As Christmas approached, I welcomed the change in pace. It was holiday time, it was summer, and I was looking forward to 1st January, 2017. Like my birthday, it meant 2016 was over and the year I was diagnosed would finally be behind me. I would never have to live that time again. My 'leap year' would be over forever.

I wasn't sad to see the year end—it was a year I would never forget—but I had big plans for 2017 and I was eager to see the clock strike twelve.

I read an article recently about 'The Santa Project', which is a movement to keep the story of Santa alive. It is really sweet, and made me think about how as children, the magic of Christmas is awesome, and as we grow up and become adults, somehow that magic leaves us. I love that there is now a National Believe Day. How fabulous to have a day dedicated to making Christmas wishes.

I personally love this time of year, with all the beautifully decorated Christmas trees, homemade wreaths, gingerbread, Christmas music, Christmas lilies and their heavenly smell, the film 'Love Actually' (I cannot tell you how many times I have seen that film!), and of course, Santa Claus.

But Christmas for me is mainly about family. We come together to share our love for one another, to share stories, to share a glass of wine (or two!), and to exchange our gifts knowing that we have just the perfect thing for our loved ones.

I was still visiting the oncology ward for my Herceptin treatment, but thankfully my specialist appointments were now every six weeks instead of three. I was finally starting to get a resemblance of a life back. My weeks were not consumed by cancer treatment anymore; I wasn't constantly reminded of my status as a cancer patient. It was liberating, I was coming out the other side. I never thought I would get to that point, that place. After months of inner turmoil, instability, and confusion, the storm clouds had passed.

I couldn't believe how strong I had been, I was tougher than I thought, I was practically invincible. My body had been through so much and I had survived. I guess I was a cancer survivor. I loathe that saying too; it conjures up another reality TV programme. I really need to think of some better words for 'journey' and 'survivor'—in fact they should be banned from cancer literature altogether.

> *"I've had to learn how to let go of my life before cancer and truly embrace and be grateful for the life I have now."*
> *– Jane Delahay*

*Tuscany*

## CHAPTER 25

It was only a week until l was leaving for the trek. Wow, that time had flown by. Of course, I had a whole lot of other things going on in my life and I really hadn't given the trek much thought at all. I hadn't even looked at where I was going to be walking or practiced speaking any Italian phrases; I suspect I would want to know how to order a glass of vino sometime during my travels.

I was nervous and excited at the same time. Nervous for the fact I knew none of my travelling companions, and excited to be going back to Italy, to see part of the country I had never been to before and see it as the locals do, on foot.

What was it going to be like, meeting all of those women who had been through the same roller coaster a cancer diagnosis gives you? Would I be similar to them? Would I even like any of them? Would they be my kind of people? What had these women been through?

God, I hope that we don't talk about cancer all the time—that will be totally depressing.

I have always been OK meeting new people and talking about the weather or interest rates, but this was different. I already thought they were my kin, these women and I shared one thing—a big thing—we had all had breast cancer. They, more than anyone I had in my family or friendship network, had experienced the same as me, the absolute same.

It was a comforting feeling. I needed to spend time with people who just got it, who totally knew the maelstrom of emotions I had experienced. I was looking forward to meeting those amazing women.

The very first person I met from the trek is a beautiful and sophisticated soul. I liked her instantly; small in stature but big on laughs and wit. She emitted that kind of world traveller panache and elegance, style and grace are two words to describe her, because it didn't matter what she wore, she always looked so stylish. How do people do that? Just throw a few things together and look fantastic? On our trek she somehow still looked fashionable in walking pants and big chunky shoes. She had a glamorous backpack—hard to imagine I know—but hers looked like a small handbag, not the big solid and unyielding thing I had.

The first day I met her she was wearing a gorgeous light blue leather jacket she had picked up in Rome on her way to Florence to meet us all on the trek. It was a very striking colour, one I had never seen before in a leather jacket, and it matched her outfit perfectly. I, on the other hand, was wearing jeans and a parka, a bright blue one that was too big for me because I had borrowed it. I had been a bit too stingy to buy a decent trekking parka but this one made me look like 'second hand Rose'. I had so many lovely jackets at home, but because I was also being stingy on the luggage space too, I didn't bring any of them.

I certainly didn't look like I could afford the hotel I was staying in. It was really very posh, the type that has turn down chocolates and complimentary slippers. I certainly made use of the slippers; I didn't pack any of those either due to small hand luggage constraints.

As it happened, I was staying in the same hotel as her for the first two nights before we met up with everyone else. She had a shopping trip on her agenda and I was happy to tag along. I am usually not the biggest shopper but something about those tiny laneways and cobblestone streets with the smell of leather in the air seemed rather nice.

We set off the next morning for a day of sightseeing and shopping. It was a rather dreary day; it had been raining most of the day before and still hadn't let up. It wasn't exactly the spring weather I was expecting, but hey, I was in Florence and about to embark on an amazing adventure.

Florence is a major draw card for tourists and it is easy to see why. In fact, Florence attracts thirteen million visitors a year—staggering! I did feel that quite a lot of them were standing in the queue to go into the cathedral and Duomo—it's free to get in, so that probably had a bearing on the crowds, too.

The cathedral is an impressive building in the middle of the city dazzling in colour with its decorative mix of green, pink, and white marble, and is the fourth largest cathedral in the world. We passed by it several times as we meandered our way through the crowds and the small streets with our umbrellas and shopping bags.

We chose to do some of the smaller churches in the outer parts of town, and proceeded to follow our map to the city walls and visit not only a few historic sites, but also a bakery the concierge had told us about that morning.

We walked and walked and ended up at the edge of town with no sign of the church we were looking for. We were certainly getting in some extra training for the trek but it was past lunchtime and we were lost and hungry. We stopped a group of girls in the street, pointed to our map, and they told us we were going in the exact opposite direction of where we wanted to go.

We laughed; off to a good start! We muddled around and finally found the place where we had the most delicious pizza I had eaten in a long time.

As we sat there watching the streams of local people coming in for their lunch, we started to talk about ourselves.

She said, "it's such a pain getting cancer, and totally inconvenient!"

She hit the nail on the head. What a pain in the arse cancer is, no one wants it, no one puts their hand up for that. She had been diagnosed nearly five years ago. She was moving on and it wasn't part of her life anymore. It was over, and as far as she was concerned, never coming back, so why talk about it? I agreed. I didn't want to talk about it either.

The weather was turning and the rain was starting to come down in sheets, so we headed back to our hotel to stay in for the night. We headed to the bar, which was in the middle of a small pond-like fountain towards the back of reception. I am not sure what purpose this water feature had, but it was pleasant and made us feel somewhat more like we were on the Italian Riviera, rather than in a hotel in Florence on a dark, rainy night.

My fellow trekker had travelled down from Rome with another member of our group. I had yet to meet her and we agreed that we should invite her over to our hotel for dinner. Tuscan white bean soup was on the menu and we didn't fancy going out in the rain again. She arrived to find us already comfortable with a few Prosecco's under our belt. As soon as she found us and we said our hellos she burst into tears.

On route to us in the rain she had stopped at an ATM to withdraw money she would need for the trek. She was harassed at the ATM by a man who tried to rob her. He stood over her while she was withdrawing money, and tried to grab her. It was a very frightening start to her holiday in Italy and she was overcome with fear. She explained another man who was inside the shop adjacent to the ATM had seen what was happening and ran to assist her. So in one foul swoop she had the very worst and the very best of human nature. She was shaken but it ended well. She had all her money, new-found friends, and a determined sense that nothing was going to stop her from having the time of her life.

Saying that, our next day travelling to the meeting point of the trek didn't actually start that well. The three of us arrived to a rather nondescript and ageing (and not in a romantic Byzantine way) hotel on a bustling Florence street.

The reception was manned by a gruff old Italian man who probably should not have been working in hospitality. I realised it was a family run business as his daughter popped out from behind the dusty fake flower arrangement to assist us with our reservations.

The floor was dirty with footsteps of rain sodden shoes (including my own), and droplets of water littering the old linoleum. I was cold, wet, and still jet lagged, and it was not really the reception I was expecting. As I dragged my suitcase around to the holding area, I noticed the sound of Australian accents and a small group of women standing in what I assumed was the breakfast room.

It was a tiny room in the centre of the reception area with square plastic tables, hard lino seats, and a small spray of fake flowers adorning the centre. It smelt musty and was far from the vision I had of cosy and stylish Italian hotels. I wanted to go back to the hotel I had stayed in the last two nights.

Beyond the strange quadrangle of a breakfast room was a huge conference room with twenty chairs all set in a circle like a camp fire, but without the fire, obviously. The room was huge, it echoed, in fact. I realised that room was where we were all to meet for our 6pm welcome and catch up. There were no tables, no drinks, no food, no welcome dinner, just chairs. If that was the standard to be expected for the rest of the trek, I was concerned.

The accommodation was one-star at best; the facilities were non-existent and the rooms had a dormitory feel about them—and not in a fun school camp way.

The meeting room was dark but bright at the same time. Blinding fluorescents and the dull glow of the street lights outside gave it an eerie vibe. I am by no means a snob when it comes to accommodation, I have stayed in some really fantastic places over the years, from one star to five, but this was just depressing. All my expectations had flown out of the dirt-smeared windows.

It was time to sit down and introduce ourselves. I scanned the room, taking in each face of the nineteen women and one man. They were all shapes and sizes, in varying degrees of a jet lagged state but smiling, and by all accounts very happy to be there.

The room all of a sudden became lively, electric in a way. I could feel the buzz of the others, with the impending excitement of starting our trek. A sense of ease came over me—I was going to get on famously with those women.

They were all smiling, eager to tell their story to us all. I was eager too; I wanted to get to know them, I suddenly became quite overcome by the enormity of what we were about to do.

One of the ladies in her introduction said, "I want to live a fearless life."

Her words resonated with me. Yes, that was it. Live fearlessly. Tomorrow, we were going to start walking 100 kilometres through Tuscany—it was a once in a lifetime experience. I was there, in Florence, about to embark on an amazing adventure.

It took about an hour to get around the room with everyone introducing themselves. I hadn't been in a situation like that since my first day of high school, but it was motivating to be part of such a diverse group of women who shared a common bond. I realised after everyone had spoken I was indeed channelling Isaac Newton, "If I have seen further, it is by standing on the shoulders of giants."

The energy in the room was totally overwhelming; everyone's story was so uplifting, so amazingly positive even for some of the group who were fighting metastatic breast cancer. People talk about cancer patients as being brave, and that room of people proved it. Totally inspiring and not for one second did they feel sorry, angry, shocked, or sad about their cancer diagnosis. It had changed their lives, and for the better, not for the worst. Breast cancer doesn't discriminate and you only had to look around the room to see that.

"Such amazing and wonderful women, who don't let the dreaded 'C' word dictate life, but live it fully every day. I am so grateful that it brought us together and I feel truly blessed." My fellow trekker will not mind me quoting her; I felt exactly the same way.

## CHAPTER 26

Day one and we were on our way; I was happy to leave the rather unsavoury accommodation behind us and was secretly hoping that it wasn't the standard I would have to get used to for the next ten days.

We were like a gaggle of geese, all talking and wandering about the footpath with our wheelie suitcases criss-crossing on our way to the bus that was to take us to our first destination, Lucca, where we would meet our local Italian guide.

Our main team leader for the trek had already introduced himself to us. He had led over twelve adventures, including climbing Kilimanjaro and running the London Marathon, and was currently based in the UK. We weren't quite climbing Everest, but it would be long days and there was a very good likelihood we would be nursing sore feet and blisters at the end of the day. He was a seasoned traveller and by all accounts quite capable of looking after twenty menopausal women.

Right from the start we knew he was someone special. It would take someone special to look after twenty women who have either had breast cancer, or supported someone with it. It was no ordinary trek. He was whimsical and energetic, but firm and fair in his instruction on how the days were to play out. Absolutely no one was allowed to be late, that was his mantra. "Be on time."

I was OK with it as I am a stickler for being on time too. For others, it took some getting used to. Some days it really was like 'browns cows' and he was farmer Brown, albeit a farmer in fancy red shorts.

But it was so much fun being in a group of like-minded people. I felt young again. It was like school camps with all your besties, it had only been a day but I was in love with them all. They came from so many walks of life, some town folk, some country folk, some on farms, and some in the happening suburbs of Sydney and Melbourne. We had an amazing cross section of locations in Australia; each person had more than just their breast cancer story to tell. These women represented the very best of all Australians, a fighting spirit and a can do attitude. It was addictive.

I found myself thinking back to the early days of my diagnosis and how I felt about it all, and how I wished I had these women around me then. I realised how important it was to share how I felt, to talk about it, to really be aware of the thoughts I was having and that I wasn't alone in thinking the way I did. It was enlightening and cathartic to be amongst those women.

The first morning in Lucca was our time to spend how we wanted. I suspected it was the tour guide's way of getting us to know each other better, which I wasn't complaining about. I was really happy to find out more about everyone.

Lucca is an extraordinary little town in Northern Tuscany; it still has its old city walls that encircle the ancient architecture hidden inside. On top of these walls is a grassy park, and we headed straight for the trail so we could get a birds eye view of the gorgeous Gothic buildings that are remarkably still intact.

The walk around the city walls is nearly four kilometres; if we were going to get used to walking, that was a good start. I spent the first hour walking with one of my new-found trekkers and I instantly liked her.

She had been under forty when she was diagnosed and had to immediately think about whether she wanted children. Breast cancer isn't supposed to happen to young women.

It is something I thought too, but the incidence of young women diagnosed with breast cancer is more common than people talk about. They face many different issues to older women, it can be a very different disease for them and more difficult to treat.

What an awful situation to be in. You are still in shock after being told you have breast cancer, and then to be told that you must harvest your eggs for future use because the treatment will kill them off. You don't even know at that point in your life if you want children but you have to make the decision quickly, and consent to more invasive surgery. She also faced the prospect of more long-term complications from treatment and had to stop taking Tamoxifen because it was wreaking all sorts of havoc on her.

I found myself becoming quite teary. I have two beautiful children whom I love more than anything, to be possibly denied that gift because you have cancer is heartbreaking.

She is just amazing, her take on her diagnosis is poignant, sensible, but also heartfelt. "I might not have the biggest scar, but the impact it had on me psychologically and physically cannot be expressed. Cancer is a presence in my daily life, hoping like hell it will never return, doing what I can to raise awareness, raising money for others, supporting and helping others through their diagnosis and treatments, but the scars...they are the biggest reminders of so many things about life, staring at me every day, they are real."

They are the untold stories; they are the reason I was there, why I had fund-raised for this worthy charity, why I wanted to start writing, to tell stories and not just my own. I was here to be the author for all those amazing and beautiful women, I was sure of it, and I had a lot to say.

Standing in the midday sunshine, in the town of Lucca, I could see that I was falling in love, falling in love with Italy. What a wondrous corner of the world this is. Tuscany in springtime, I honestly thought I had died and gone to heaven.

Lucca and its surrounds are steeped in history and tradition, and its central location in Italy allowed it to be a prosperous hub trade for centuries. The Via Francigena - the great Medieval pilgrimage route along which lie villages, castles, abbeys and parish churches – we were set to travel the same pilgrim path; the tiny little signs of the pilgrim man and his swag over his shoulder were everywhere, a simple symbol of perseverance.

It was an apt description of us, too. Twenty women on a pilgrimage of self-discovery. That small pilgrim became quite a comforting sign as we embarked on our trip of a lifetime.

As we neared the end of our shaded walk courtesy of the side walk trees in and around the city walls in Lucca, we spied a carousel. The old fashioned type, with dancing horses, wild animals, lights and festoons, and the beautiful sounds of childhood.

Our eyes brightened. "Let's go on the carousel!"

We all jumped at the chance to be foolish, to be childish, to have fun. Wasn't that what this was all about?

We chose our horses; they had beautiful plumes in their necks and were painted so perfectly. We were the only ones on it, just us, the crazy Australian women who were squealing with delight, riding around and around the carousel. What fun. I was beginning to think I had a lot more in common with them than breast cancer. To top off the fun we were having, a gelato was in order. We piled the cones up high from the self-service machines that were dispensing the most amazing creations of ice cream I had seen in my life. Mango and lemon, yes please!

We had such a fun day. I felt like a child; no responsibilities, no one but me to worry about, and a bunch of new-found friends. I couldn't be happier.

We made our way back to our accommodation for our nightly briefing. It was a mandatory meeting, and we were to talk about the next day's activities and when and how we were to start the trek.

It was time to meet our local Italian guide, and I am not sure what I was expecting, but he wasn't it. He was much younger than us, and with his wild Einstein hair and round framed glasses he looked more like a dishevelled University student than an adventure guide armed with the responsibility of looking after us all on a five day hike. But he was all smiles and spoke the most fascinating broken English, which would in the next five days be the cause of misunderstanding, laughter, and mayhem. He explained our route and where it would take us, and touched on the level of fitness we were going to need to accomplish it.

I was starting to wonder if I had indeed done enough training. Well, too late now, anyway. I was there and I was going to give it a good crack.

Our local guide summed up the trek and assured us we would have the time of our lives. He ordered a round of Aperol Spritz—how civilised, how Italian!

At that moment two bicycles rode past, two women, in at least their eighties, with high heeled shoes and flowing skirts. How amazing, and again, how Italian!

I am going to love being here. I just know it.

## CHAPTER 27

I awoke the next morning, early and eager to get started. It was too early for breakfast so I decided to take a walk in the morning glow. I decided I would bring a journal to write notes in about my travels (glad I did, they are all in this book!). I hadn't started and pulled out page one. I walked a short distance to the Piazza San Martino and sat on the stairs from where I could see the back of the church of San Giovanni and Santa Reparta. The bright blue sky, the clean smell of the morning air, the birds singing in chorus, the magnificent monuments that humans have built, the details of the facades, the trees with their curly leaves. Just being.

The rumble of a lorry over the cobble stones interrupted my solitude and I looked up to see the back of a black figure coming out of the church. It was a nun. She had her head down looking at her smart phone—that made me giggle, she was so modern and old world at the same time.

On our last walk around Lucca, we visited the Lucca Cathedral. Embedded in the right pier of the portico is the Labyrinth maze dated from the 12th or 13th century. Our guide said the maze has significance and the mythology says, "You may never get to the middle but it is not about reaching that, it is about finding your way through the maze, the maze of life and going the wrong way is all about learning from our mistakes and that course correction is sometimes necessary."

I like that very much. Even the wrong direction is the right direction when we need to take that particular path.

It was time to leave and finally get started for the reason we were all there. With back packs on, water filled, lunch packed, and walking poles ready, we were off. From the moment we entered the Tuscan countryside, I was mesmerised. I had never seen anything quite so beautiful in my life. Wild red poppies littered the trail and the meadows, their wobbling heads swaying in the morning breeze and their vibrant colour dotting the scenery. The grass was so green it was an emerald colour—nothing like our burnt grass in Australia—lush and almost luminous. My heart jumped, I was witnessing something so beautiful I nearly cried. That was living in the moment. That was literally stopping to smell the roses, to be in the now. I was drinking in the feeling of being in the present and I now know what it really means.

Well, there I was in the middle of Tuscany realising my own power of now and it was exhilarating. I was going to enjoy every minute of it. I think I finally got what it was all about; live for now, right now, right here in the most amazing place. In my mind, I was at peace. I could see it, I had everything in me and more, I had all I needed. It was huge. I could see clearly (for the rain had gone). I had a purpose, could feel it. I was overwhelmed and tears welled up in my eyes.

I could barely explain it. It was the joy of the beautiful landscape, it was the camaraderie I felt from my fellow trekkers and it was literally life changing. I had arrived at that wonderful place, completely at peace. At peace with what I had endured for twelve months. I wasn't afraid anymore. I could do this; I could be an inspiration to others and myself.

That path has been called many things, but I like the saying 'divine storm'. Translated I could see the meaning of it: 'God's disturbance'. My life had been disturbed violently, I had had my own thunderstorms, my own lightning, my own snow, but after the rain comes a rainbow. I was standing there, basking in that thought, all those beautiful colours sprinkling down on me. I had come through the storm.

As we wound our way through sandy paths, tree lined roads, and vineyards, the sun was rising high in the sky and the blue hue became more vivid. Our group became the long snake of a walking group. It was inevitable that we would all be walking at different paces due to us all having different fitness levels.

I was nowhere near the front of the pack, nor the back. Just meandering in the middle, going at a relaxed pace. I didn't want to rush the experience. We formed small groups along the trail, finding our kin and walking and talking at the same time. I wanted to spend time with everyone; I wanted to get to know my fellow travellers even if it was just for a few minutes as we stopped to let the stragglers catch up. I was fascinated by everyone's story, they were so different from mine, but at the same time so similar.

I totally hit the jackpot when I was paired with my roommate for the trek. I had opted for the shared accommodation; it was cheaper and I liked the fact I would share with someone I didn't know. I hoped it would be like school camp, where you shared stories of the day and generally had fun, ate sweets, and giggled. I got that and more.

My roommate had been sent from heaven. We were the perfect match. Even to the point where other people thought we already knew each other from before the trek. We didn't, but we knew as soon as met that we were kindred spirits.

My roommate was younger than me by nearly ten years and she

is a single mum, which alone is worthy of praise and honour—that is a tough job without being diagnosed with breast cancer too. No one could imagine what it would be like to be the sole parent of a gorgeous child and wonder what fate awaits you after finding out you have cancer. If people knew the inner struggles and feeling of total despair about the future of your family after a cancer diagnosis, they would think twice about complaining about their infected toenail.

Her laugh was infectious—she giggled like a school girl about anything. She always had a smile on her face, always. The room lit up in her presence, her spirit was unfathomable, she was so determined to do this trek, she had planned it for nearly twelve months, and she was not going to miss out on anything; a sentiment I shared. We weren't going to come to the other side of the world and not experience everything we possibly could, we not only walked the entire trek, we did all of the town walking tours, ate all of the food put in front of us, and tried many variations of Aperol and Lemoncello. I loved at the end of the day I could go back to my room and she was either already there, or by my side walking the hotel hallways. We truly shared the experience together.

Our rooms were usually configured with two single beds; I am not sure of the size of a European single bed, but the majority of them seemed quite short. My feet inevitably hung over the edge. Another fellow trekker likened the beds to what might be in a nun's room. Suffice to say they were small and narrow.

If by chance we had one single bed and one double bed, my roommate would always be happy for me to take the bigger bed, which was so gracious. On those nights I would sleep horizontally across the bed. We would lay there and just natter in the semi darkness. We talked about our day and our lives, it was therapeutic. I never tired of her conservations about her life in country NSW and stories of her gorgeous daughter—we had that in common, beautiful girls in our lives.

After several failed surgeries to get clear margins around her initial tumour, my roommate had a double mastectomy. No reconstruction, my roommate has no breasts. Think about that for a minute. Think about how totally devastating it would be to lose both of your breasts and have a flat chest with scars where your breasts used to be. There is brave, and then there is brave. She is the latter. To be faced with the reality before the age of forty is something most of us will never have to contemplate, and there she was walking 100 kilometres though the Tuscan countryside. There was no stopping her.

Those women were not resting on their laurels. They are doers and thinkers, women to aspire to be, women who know what tough is, women who never give up, not even for one minute. They don't complain, they just get on with it. I felt humbled in their company and more so in the company of my roommate. I never heard her even complain about the accommodation (and sometimes there were definitely things to complain about). She saw life through rose coloured glasses; everything is glamorous, wonderful, and marvellous. What a way to see the world, to be the beacon of positive, it was hard not to happy around her. She has climbed many mountains mentally and she still has a smile upon her face.

That is a lesson for us all right there.

Our first day of trekking took us from San Miniato to Gambassi Terme, the terrain followed a trail through oak and chestnut woods, vineyards, and olive groves. That is the Tuscan landscape we are all familiar with. Quintessential Italy, and it was putting on a damn fine display. Wide open spaces, green rolling hills, tiny little medieval hill top towns with amazing architecture, cobbled stone walls and paths, we traversed it all and it was nothing short of spectacular. I was filled with energy and vitality after a day's walking, I couldn't wait to get to the next destination and order an Aperol Spritz (it had become my new favourite alcoholic drink, along with a few other members of the team—including our guide). He said it was never too early for an Aperol Spritz!

When my roommate and I arrived at our next hotel we were told there was no room for us. No room at the inn, just like Mary and Joseph.

"But that's okay," our Italian guide explained. "The owner of this hotel has an apartment in the village that you can sleep in tonight."

Our accommodation had gotten slightly better since Florence—at least two-stars—but now we being shuffled into a tiny Fiat Panda to be whisked away from our fellow trekkers to someone's house. I was very glad I wasn't on my own, it was quite the most bizarre thing, and we seemed to be going out of town from where we had just been.

We were still in our sweaty trekking gear, desperate for a shower, and it looked like we were going to be staying miles away. After circling the town for what seemed like forever, we arrived in a piazza in front of a very large wooden door.

"Here's the keys," the driver said, then took off and left us standing alone in a very handsome looking village square. Nonetheless, we were rather perplexed.

We opened the huge wooden double doors that opened up to a very large dark foyer with a staircase leading upstairs. It was quite reminiscent of the inside of a castle, the type you visit as a child where it is dark, musty, and just a tiny bit freaky. Thank goodness no skeletons fell out of the cupboards near the stairs.

As we hauled our suitcases upstairs we realised it wasn't too bad after all. Yes, it was someone's home, but it was clean, tidy, and quite quaint in a renovated medieval way.

No sooner had we dumped our bags on the bed, my roommate

announced she had locked her padlock keys inside her case. Oops, everything was locked in her bag. No secret openings, no spare keys, aside from cutting her bag open we had to come up with a solution. After walking twenty kilometres and getting the run around with our accommodation, it was not the scenario we were envisaging. There were drinks awaiting, beautiful Italian food awaiting. She couldn't even have a shower and change her underpants!

OK, let's figure this out, I thought. Bobby pin, check!

We twisted and turned the bobby pin inside the lock barrel for half an hour, to no avail. We would make terrible thieves; we couldn't get the catch to click. Looked like it might require a pair of scissors to cut through the fabric to get to the keys. At that point, my roommate admitted it wasn't her case and if she cut it open she would have to replace it, which wasn't ideal. She encouraged me to head off for my shower and then at least one of us would be ready for aperitif hour. When I emerged from my shower she looked like the Cheshire cat; she had done it, she had picked the lock.

I think she could have a new career as a thief after all.

After all the kerfuffle we finally got to the restaurant for dinner and it blew our minds. Wow, the place was amazing. Set in gardens a few kilometres out of town, I will name it here because it is so fabulous: Tattoria Toscana Sant'llario.

I had gone from vinyl seats and plastic tablecloths in Florence, to five star dining in a matter of days. What a turnaround, and I couldn't be happier tasting the local Italian cuisine and drinking the wine straight from the local vineyards I had walked past during the day. What a way to end the day—I could get used to that.

I had gotten to know quite a few of my fellow trekkers quite well by now. There was a group of six of us that really bonded. We were like a group of teenagers, giggling, incessantly chatting, eating and drinking, and having the time of our lives. One member of the six was seventy, yes. Seventy years old. She is as old as my mum and as much as I love my mum, I could not see her doing a hundred kilometre walk. It blew my mind. Not only was she doing the trek she is a dragon boater too, representing Australia. Now that is an achievement in itself without having had breast cancer to add to the equation.

She was frightfully funny; her dry sense of humour was a welcome relief when walking up very steep hills. Her phrases of 'just a little rise' were her way of letting us know we had a large hill to climb, so get ready. Her walking poles would clicker clack on the path behind us; she was everyone's team buddy. The vocal one, the one who told jokes, and generally kept us all light-hearted when we were huffing and puffing up the hills. If she could do it, so could we. She was the benchmark, the yardstick, the elder, the one who we all looked up to and wanted to emulate. I totally want to be like her at seventy, still climbing hills and poking fun at life, she is a woman after my own heart.

As we meandered down the walking trail the sun was high in the sky and the clouds were like pillows dotted against the blue. We turned the corner and I could see in the distance, popping out of absolutely nowhere, the splendour of San Gimignano and its skyline of bell towers.

I mean, wow! I had read about the mediaeval town but nothing prepares you for the majesty of the place. San Gimignano is a UNESCO (United Nations Educational, Scientific and Cultural Organisation) World Heritage site. The families who controlled the town back in the 11th to 13th centuries, (that history itself is hard to even contemplate) built around seventy-two tower houses as symbols of their power and wealth. Although only fourteen towers survive, they stand out from kilometres away like an inspiration from a children's theme park, glorious and symbolic in their appearance.

The Via Franciegna crosses the entire town, from one city wall gate on one side, to the other. The town grew around two primary squares, the Piazza della Cisterna and the Piazza Duomo. The first, after an octagonal travertine (a form of limestone frequently used for building in Italy), well was laid in 1273. The structure dominates the square, it is the centrepiece of the most harmonious array of ancient buildings. It was picture postcard worthy, and I couldn't take my eyes off it. It was quite magnificent and nothing like I had ever seen in my life. It is totally untransformed with modern life; standing in the town centre was like taking a trip back in time, if you closed your eyes you could imagine life there in the Middle Ages; a perfect little town with ornate walls, beautiful monuments, and a double town wall to keep it all within the town precinct. A perfect centre of architecture and Italianisms, how grand. I was mesmerised.

San Gimignano has so many little cobblestone alleyways, arches, churches, piazzas, that it was easy to get lost, and I did. It is a very ancient city, but tucked away in lovely little shop fronts are some pretty good shopping if you are after the local produce. There are incredible cheese shops, the typical Tuscan cheese is Pecorino and we had already had several dinners which included this very tasty cheese. Although it has a pretty strong aromatic flavour and smell.

It was possible to smell the cheese shops before you arrived at them. The cheese shops I saw were very handsome indeed, almost like a posh department store food hall, beautiful glass cabinets full of delicious cheese, and the cheese mongers were very happy to hand out samples.

There was also local olive oil available, which I would have loved to have brought home but the thought of a glass bottle of olive oil exploding in my suitcase put me off. That was not something I would want to explain to border force.

We were so fortunate to be staying right in the Piazza della Cisterna. When I arrived in our room, I couldn't believe it; I had what must be the best view ever from a hotel room. The window outlined the view back over where we had just walked up to the city walls and over the rolling hills of Tuscany. How lucky I was, I could have sat there staring at that view all day.

But on to important things. Our guide told us there in San Gimignano was the world's best gelato. After a long day trekking it sounded perfect. I have never seen so many flavours in a gelato shop. There was lavender, champagne, espresso, ginger, and some of the combinations were incredible (and some not for the faint hearted!). Lychee and rose, saffron and pinenuts, raspberry and rosemary (I tried that one and it was so delicious). As we sat enjoying our world famous gelato in a world famous site, it was not lost on me that I was indeed living a life that twelve months ago had seemed impossible.

Our local guide told us he would take us on an impromptu walking tour of the city and show us some of the famous artworks and churches, but two of my fellow trekkers decided that they would take a quick trip to Volterra instead, which was nearby and famed for the Twilight movies. They were both big fans of the movie and given we were so close didn't want to miss the opportunity to see where their handsome vampire hero had visited in the movie. I remembered the scene in the movie and though it would be quite something to see, I was happy to do the more sedate walking tour of the Italian art masterpieces in San Giminanao and possibly another round of gelato.

I was keen to hear about their escapades to a neighbouring town of significance and was waiting for them to return with their stories. As it turns out, the fountain the main heroine runs through was not actually in the main square of Volterra, it had apparently been built for the movie and was no longer there. That was disappointing for them, but they enjoyed all the other film locations that are actually still there, including the Palazzo dei Priori Clock Tower. My fellow trekkers told me in fact Montepulciano (another 110 kilometres away) is where many of the scenes were filmed. They did not have enough time to visit there too. Well, maybe next time.

It was time to say goodbye to San Gimignano, I absolutely loved being there and instantly fell in love with the beautiful town that dominates the Tuscan countryside. I could have stayed there for days just wandering the cobblestoned streets and soaking in its beauty.

Next, we were on our way to Colle di Val D'Elsa taking us through olive groves and cypress avenues. That marked half way through our trek. It was hard to believe, I felt like it was going too fast. I wanted the experience to last longer, I felt so at peace there with my trekking comrades and the scenery was beyond beautiful. Quietly walking through the magnificent hills was so soul nourishing. Being outdoors in the smiling sun, the blue skies that went forever… it was magic.

We arrived in Colle di Val D'Elsa earlier in the day than previous towns even though it was a pretty intense walk. The hills were very steep and the last rise up to the town was practically vertical. By that stage we had lost a few of our fellow walkers—not actually lost them—but they had to sit out of the day's walking. We had eleven of the twenty on the walk, it was a much smaller group.

It was still amazing and the town was as picturesque as you could get. I was glad I didn't miss it and felt for the team members who did. But it was a tough day's walk; we had three hill climbs in total and two river crossings. The pictures we took from the hill top town are some of my favourites. They give the real scale of the countryside and the warm terracotta buildings glowed in the spring sun, giving it the rich air of sumptuousness.

I was glad to give my legs a break and took the opportunity of arriving early to hit the town centre palazzo and find a bar that served Aperol Spritz—a big one.

We headed for the Piazza Arnolfo de Cambio in the town centre, a beautiful palazzo with a massive fountain smack bang in the middle. It was a warm day and the square was humming with people all in search of a lazy afternoon.

That brings me to the Italian siesta. It was something I did know about but had completely forgot when I arrived in Italia. We found ourselves in deserted town centres between the hours of 1pm and 4pm, every day. Shop doors closed, grills lowered with signs turned to signal that siesta had started. The feint noises from the back of those stores were the only signs of life from many shopping strips. Occasionally, you could smell cooking wafts emanating from gardens at the back of the palazzos.

There was something quite genial and sociable about a siesta. I am a fan. I wondered why the Italians drank wine at lunchtime because I know it would put me to sleep. But that is exactly why—they can sleep! It's actually very civilised and I think that we should adopt it worldwide, I'm sure there wouldn't be as many stressed out people. The Italians I met on my Tuscan travels were so laid back, relaxed, and enjoying life. Just as it should be.

Our lives are too fast paced, too crazy, no wonder we are mentally fatigued, mentally ill. We don't take time out to be with family, cook delicious meals, and rest a little. We are our own worst enemies. We worry too much about making money, and not about sacrificing that time to just 'be'.

One morning when I was out early looking for a decent coffee, I ran into our local Italian guide. Hair a mess, and looking slightly dishevelled, I thought he may just have slept in his clothes. He quite honestly said that in Italy a black coffee and a cigarette was the breakfast of champions; I must say I did partake in the coffee and the cigarette.

    I had to giggle, it was probably how thousands of Italians started their day and I don't blame them, how fabulous. The slower pace of life is comforting; there is something quite lovely about taking a conscious break, taking time out from the hustle and bustle, finding that place of respite in yourself. It is a time to enjoy and do anything but work; it's about family and food, two very important features of Italian life. La Famiglia, I love that word.

# CHAPTER 28

Every night (or sometimes mornings), I wrote in my journal. It is something I started many months before, something I was loathe to do at first, but I found a certain solace in it thanks to Ruby.

When I first started writing to myself, I wrote all sorts of stuff. But it was changing. I wrote about so many things that were not always positive, but I wasn't putting myself down anymore. I was noticing what happened around me, everyday things I had barely noticed in the past.

I had never stopped to hear water flowing down a river, leaves swaying and rustling in the breeze. I actually became aware of the sounds in my world; it was like I had picked up a sixth sense. I practiced yoga every morning of the trek in my pyjamas on any bit of floor I could find in the hotel room; sometimes that was very little.

My roommate would often wake with me squished into a corner with my legs up on the wall. She decided a few mornings into the trek to join me, she was a novice at yoga, but very keen to understand more. To be honest she was probably tired of me banging on about the benefits of yoga and disrupting her sleep at 6am in the morning too. We did a few poses together and some breathing exercises. One morning I said to her, "in the stillness you can hear sounds you have never really heard. I know it seems a bit cuckoo but it's true, still your mind and you will hear joy."

That morning we heard birds chirping and my roommate said, "I have never heard such a beautiful noise."

But here's the thing, birds sing around us every day we just don't hear them. We don't take the time out to be aware of how many exquisite things live with us on this planet. Every day I get outside into nature and just soak it in. It's exhilarating, and over time that practice has helped me overcome the demons swirling around in my head, I guess it became my kind of mindfulness. Sometimes we just need to be silent.

It was around that time on the trek I met a woman who I can only describe as a warrior. What a woman! I had never met anyone like her before. It had taken me a few days to talk to her because I truly didn't know what to say to her. She has metastatic breast cancer—it is not curable.

Her early breast cancer was the same as mine, she had similar treatments to me, but hers had come back. And it had come back in her bones. She calls it her 'hitch-hiker', but no one stops to pick up a hitch-hiker like cancer. She is one of a kind, a truly courageous spirit she has chutzpah by the bucket loads.

## CHAPTER 29

Every person who has had breast cancer lives with the fear of it coming back. While the survival rates are at an all-time high in Australia, there is still a very small chance it will return. I try not to dwell on that aspect of the disease. I focus on the 90% chance it won't come back, not the 10% that it will. It's not easy some days, but I have been able to manage the fear through all of the techniques I have learnt over the past twelve months. I don't beat myself up for thinking about it, instead I use the cloud analogy, 'clouds are just thoughts', they pass.

I had met a few women in the chemotherapy unit that had metastatic cancer but I didn't know them well. I think at the time I just skirted around the subject because it was too scary to talk about. I thought that if I said too much it might rub off on me—crazy I know—but at the time, I didn't want to be there and their situation was scaring me senseless. I had not even digested my own diagnosis, let alone have understanding and compassion to spare for them. It was too much to take in. I barely understood the new cancer world I had entered and incurable cancer was just another level of scary. It was beyond my comprehension.

I wanted to talk to her, because she had this air of mysteriousness and a tough exterior, but I could sense she had a big heart underneath the armour. I suppose it is understandable to shield yourself from others and your condition, it is only natural. It's not like you would want to stand on the rooftops and shout out the fact you have incurable cancer. You don't want the sorrow, the pity. You want people to talk to you like a real human being and not about your situation. I decided I would only talk to her about her cancer if she brought it up first.

Of all the trekkers she was the one most decked out in what I would describe as outdoor gear. She had the whole ensemble going on.

I had active wear pieces, like my walking pants, but the rest of my outfit was from a discount department store. My thoughts were that I probably wouldn't be wearing the gear again in a hurry so the less I spent on it, the better. I bought decent shoes and pants which were the business, but my tops were cheap and cheerful.

Hers was all variations of the colour pink. Bright pink, pale pink, cherry pink. It was all mix and match. I could see the point; I could see the irony, the paradox. But she looked fabulous; she was instantly recognisable in her outfits. She also had a very spiffy backpack, the best of the bunch, certainly better than my second hand one from my husband. As long as it did the job it didn't matter really but hers was like a small spaceship, I was waiting for it to do the dishes and sing songs too.

Because we were a small group on the third day, I had the chance to get to know her. We walked many kilometres that day just chatting about anything and everything. I was totally intrigued and impressed by her tattoos; she had some really amazing ones. I think it shows her rebel side, her 'I don't give a shit' attitude. I loved it. It was inspiring, and if I could just take one leaf out of her book I would be happy. What strength—and not only to endure the pain of all of those tattoos!

As we walked along we laughed, admired our beautiful

surroundings, took photos, and felt blessed we could experience such wonders and reflect on how lucky we were. We might have had cancer, and in her case still does, but we were the luckiest gals in the world to be standing in that most amazing place and we knew it.

Her 'hitch-hiker' has been behaving itself, she recently had scans that showed no new cancer activity and I could not have been more thrilled for her. She still has chemo every three weeks but it is doing its job, and she says, "I am not quite as good as new but I am probably as good as a reasonably priced second hand car." I love her. What a superstar. Beautiful new friends. I was truly blessed.

The next morning we were on our way to Monteriggioni where our route took us through the densely forested hill of Montagnole. We had only fourteen kilometres to walk, which was easier than the previous days, and I was happy to just plod along.

My legs were holding up well and I had no blisters, which I was ever so grateful for. Some trekkers had more band-aids covering their feet than skin showing, it was a sight to see and not in a good way. Blood blisters, skin falling off, big swollen parcels of skin waiting to pop pus, all rather gross and I was happy my feet had lasted the distance so far.

When we stopped for a water break or a toilet break, shoes would come off and band-aids replaced. It was almost a ritual. One aspect of the trek that actually never dawned on me until I started was going to the toilet. A pretty basic human function and we were told that there were no 'toilet stops' in the Tuscan countryside; you had to pee in the bushes. Hence the list of tissues/toilet paper to be included in your backpack, yet even then I didn't make the connection. I coined the phrase 'bear in the woods' for when anyone needed to stop for a wee.

It had been a long time since I had to go the toilet in the

outdoors; the first time I went discreetly behind a bush I peed all over my shoes.

Wow, I'm not great at this. Next time I must adjust my stance, I thought. Well, it took me nearly all week to perfect said stance and I inevitably had wet shoes every time I emerged from the bushes. Thank goodness I had bought waterproof shoes so at least I didn't have wee in my socks too. I am very grateful that the urge for a 'number two' never eventuated whilst walking the trek; I would have been in all sorts of trouble.

Those are the things you don't think about when you conjure up the beauty of walking the Tuscan countryside. How romantic and lovely to walk through the splendour, you think. Not once did I conjure up an image of trying to find a suitable spot to wee.

The walk up to Monteriggioni was staggeringly beautiful but vertical. It is situated on top of a natural hillock, a medieval walled town that was built strategically there as a defensive fort. But in 2017, whilst spectacular, it was a huge hill to climb and by the time we got to the top I had put my body through something it rarely did. I needed to sit down fast. It was by far the hardest part of the trek, and I had done it. Wow. I gave myself and my fellow trekkers a pat on the back.

As we staggered through gates of the roughly bricked walls of Monteriggioni I was transfixed. It is possibly the most beautiful little place on earth, so perfect in every way. The old city walls encircled the town like a warm hug. The fourteen towers are imposing structures all set out in perfect unison to the portals and gates at their side. It looks like an enormous medieval Lego set. The central piazza Roma is a simple square with a church, several stores selling local produce, and houses. The village as it stands is essentially the original one, the towers went through a renovation back in the 16th century but otherwise it is perfectly preserved.

There is one solitary café-come-general store, selling everything from panini's to pasta. It also sold alcohol, hallelujah! I needed a very large beer.

What I absolutely love about Italy is you can buy a large can of beer in the same fridge as a soft drink. No distinction between alcohol and non-alcoholic, it is interspersed with everything you can keep cold, including salami.

The store had two large fridges at the front that were brimming with local delicacies and I reached for two large local beers for me and my new-found friend, the seventy year old trekker.

We sat in the Piazza di Roma in our sweaty trekking clothes, and took in the extremely pleasant surroundings while pouring our beer into 500ml pilsner glasses. The sun was shining brilliant blue, the pale sand buildings were throwing afternoon shadows, and I was in bliss. That beer was possibly the best beer I had ever had, I was so parched from our walk, and water just wasn't going to suffice. It was heaven.

Our fellow trekkers headed for the gelato bar and the small stores selling local Tuscan souvenirs. I was very happy to stay there for a very long time. Our local Italian guide joined us and lit a cigarette. Oh, how nice, beer and cigarettes, that was what I call civilised.

As we chatted and enjoyed our beverages, which by this stage had grown in number to three each, we realised we had missed the transfer to the hotel. I don't actually remember the call out, I remember there were three runs to the hotel, they didn't have a mini van large enough for us all so that meant three separate trips.

That had happened often along our trail, sometimes even family members helped out with transfers. I had a particularly interesting transfer in the back of a Peugeot that I had to share with the contents of the owner's home by the look of it. Although I wasn't sure; it could have just been her usual commuting stuff. I had to be careful not to sit in the empty pizza boxes. As our Italian guide was with us, it was not too much of a drama; they certainly couldn't leave him behind, though they probably wouldn't have had the same qualms about us.

Our accommodation that night was nothing short of awesome. The Relais Borgo San Luigi is a paradise set in 60,000 square metres of Tuscan countryside. The hotel is an original 17th century building and you could lose yourself easily in the lavender and citrus tree gardens. It also had a pool.

We hadn't had that luxury yet on the trek and after a warm spring day it was just what we needed. Our guide was first to jump in, along with our eldest trekker. They were game, I thought; it was still a bit cold for me.

As we made our way down to the pool area, there was much splashing from the crowd that had descended on the pool. I pulled up a deck chair and admired my beautiful surroundings. I soaked up the ambience of the place and pretended to be rich and famous. How lovely.

As the sun was setting, a definite summer vibe arrived. At the wisteria laced pergola at the side of the pool, waiters were setting up for a party. A party, how fab! It wasn't for us.

From our viewpoint at the pool we were wondering what sort of party. A wedding? A birthday? The size of the place made it hard to know just how many people were actually there. The hotel had seventy-three rooms and I had not seen many other people, but they must be around somewhere.

As people started arriving for their welcome drinks, we worked out that they were from a company, and it was corporate function. I never found out who or where they were from, but they did know how to party.

After dinner we adjourned to the very cute little fireplace area (which would be fab in winter) and ordered a round of Prosecco.

We were joined by both our guides and huddled into two big plump sofas to chill out and enjoy ourselves and our surrounds. Not long after we heard the distinct sounds of music, loud music, in fact heavy metal music. It sort of didn't really suit the surroundings of the genial historic place but we thought hey, why not? Let's get up and dance too.

We danced around our table and the corridor to the toilet; we were jumping up and down, twirling and spinning each other around. Our guides were hilarious, two men dancing together and busting out moves that lacked agility but were fun to watch. A cross between a Russian folk dance and Austrian knee slapping is the best way to describe it. It was vaudeville, and fun, and just what we needed; to laugh until our cheeks were sore.

A representative from the corporate company approached us and asked us to come and join their party. They had been watching us jiving along to their music and must have thought we looked like a bunch of crazy Australians that might like a party. Indeed we do and we did.

We joined their team and danced in unison to ACDC's It's a long way to the top. I liked the Australian theme in the music, I am not sure if was deliberate.

We danced and danced until we were practically the only people left. We had out danced the entire party. By that stage we were slightly drunk, very sweaty, and nursing sore feet. It had started to lightly rain outside and I headed out there to cool off.

How much fun was that? I hadn't danced like that since my years at the local club in the eighties. I was exhausted really. I was forty-eight now, not twenty-eight, I wasn't up to drinking and partying all night long anymore, but gee what fun we had. My roommate very luckily had some hydralytes, which hadn't been cracked open for any reason so far. I had a reason now. She had carried around that enormous first aid kit for a week and not used a single thing in it. At least I would lighten her load by a few grams.

I awoke the next morning with rather a large hangover. My own fault of course, but I think the hydralyte did make it more bearable. I had to walk nineteen kilometres. My breakfast consisted of a can of Fanta and a cigarette—talk about breakfast of champions.

That was also the morning we would hold our 'BCNA Mini-Field of Women ceremony'. There, we stuck our pink ladies on a spike and put them into the ground, with a pink label around her neck inscribing any message you liked.

I wrote, "Go hard or go home." My feelings from the night before, I suspect.

Maybe it wasn't what they were expecting but I thought their sentiments (whilst admirable) were a tiny bit depressing. All that remembering this and that stuff. I get it, some people want to remember people who have passed away from breast cancer, but I wanted to live for now, right now. And that meant the people who are alive now. I don't take away from their memories but what we went through is not doom and gloom, it is inspiring and awesome to be there and be raising money for women who are experiencing a cancer diagnosis.

It was also a time to congratulate everyone standing there, right now. I know people don't agree with me but I stand firm, those ceremonies should be about looking forward not back. Having said that, the ceremony was moving, there were tears and hugs and a huge sense of camaraderie amongst us all. The pink ladies all standing upright on the lawn in the morning sun was quite the sight to behold, it was symbolic and had a real sense of ceremony, which was uplifting and emotional. It is apparently something BCNA does on all of the fundraising treks; the vision of the pink ladies standing tall on their spikes in all corners of the world is quite the achievement. I would just like to see more positive, and not so much negative.

I nursed my hangover for the entire morning and finally came good around lunchtime. We were on our way to Siena, our final destination. I couldn't believe it was our last day of trekking; we had walked nearly 100 kilometres, how amazing! It hadn't felt like that at all.

Siena is another UNESCO World Heritage site and one of the most visited cities in Italy. I was looking forward to arriving there but sad it was the last day I would be walking Tuscany with those beautiful women. It was a day of reflection for me. I was really proud of myself; I am not embarrassed to say I had come a long way, literally. Not just in kilometres but in my life.

I had found out so much about myself in those past fifteen months, I had always been rather sceptical of people who rush off to an ashram or go to some remote island for months on end to 'find themselves'. I get it now; finding 'me' changed my life. I am not sure exactly where and when I found myself, maybe it was in Tuscany, maybe it was at the beach, maybe in the company of friends and loved ones, or maybe it was just one day in the shower. Who knows? But I am very happy I didn't wait another forty-seven years to find out. I have so much I want to do in this thing called life.

# CHAPTER 30

Our last day trekking was jovial and reflective; I think everyone felt the same as me, very proud of our achievements on a personal level and on a fundraising level. As a team we had hit the $100,000 mark. So awesome, and there was a definite spring in our step as we patted each other on the back for our accomplishments.

The sun was shining high in the sky and as we followed the via Francigena. The wild red poppies covered the green fields for as far as the eye could see. We wore our team polos that had been designed by BCNA and we wore them proudly all day. Pink ladies in our backpacks and pink lady silhouettes emblazoned on our polos, I felt like I was in the movie Grease! We were a sea of pink on that last day of trekking, loud and proudly supporting BCNA and ourselves as cancer warrior princesses (better title than survivor!).

Our trail led us through wooded trees and the outer suburban paths of the city of Siena. Our final destination point was the city walls of Siena, and as we approached the final few hundred metres we were showered in flower confetti and cheers.

We all hugged one another and took selfies. We had done it.

We had two days in Siena to sightsee and take in the most magnificent and fascinating city. There was a lot to see, too much for two days but in the heart of Siena is the Piazza Il Campo, famous for the Palio horse race where horses run around the piazza two times every summer. We weren't there at the time of the horse race, which was disappointing because it looks absolutely amazing in the photos our guide showed us.

Standing in the middle of the piazza, I could only imagine what the roar and thunder of all of those horses must sound like and what a spectacle it must be. I could imagine people hanging out of the windows above the restaurant awnings cheering and encouraging their chosen horse to win.

It is the most glorious piazza, much larger than I expected. The most remarkable part is the shell shape square and its 'knife like' pavers, it looks like large pieces of pizza. It has nine sections outlined with little white stones that divide the pizza slices.

Rising up from the piazza is The Torre del Mangia, a very stunning tower with distinctly different levels of marble, stone and brick. It is an imposing building, and stands at eighty-eight metres high; you can see it for miles. Our Italian guide told us many curious stories about the tower, notably about a bell ringer. Its name is unusual. In Italian it roughly means, 'Tower of the Eater', apparently from a nickname of one of the first bell ringers who liked a good Italian meal (who doesn't?!) and had the task of ringing the bells on the hour, every hour.

I imagine running up all 400 stairs hourly was exhausting. But the outlook from there is pretty spectacular, as you have a bird's eye view over the entire city of Siena.

We decided we would take it easy that afternoon and park ourselves in a bar that overlooked the amazing piazza. I had met the most incredible and amazing women, each and every one of them. Some of who will be lifelong friends.

Who would have thought I would be there sitting in the most exquisite place only twelve months after my cancer diagnosis? My life had changed immeasurably in that time, to the point where my former life was unrecognisable to me. I had weathered the storm and come out the other end. I have surprised myself really. Who would ever have thought I was capable of such inner strength?

I am, in fact, quite awesome.

Self-love, I have buckets of it now. I enjoy even the smallest things, giggle to myself, smile more, and sing at the top of my voice in the car to my favourite songs. Life is full of wonderful things, they are around us each and every day, I have opened my eyes and my heart to them.

This could not have been truer; I was living proof of it. Yes, I am also a different person physically, my left breast will never look or feel the same. I have scars, war wounds, bumpy and permanently changed skin, and different coloured hair, but I am still me, and I am alive. I am here to enjoy my life on planet earth and I am going to make the most of every minute.

In fact, this minute right now, looking across the magnificent piazza in Siena, I am the luckiest girl in the world. I feel very fortunate to be sitting here with my new-found friends and enjoying life as it is meant to be. I am living proof it is never too late or you are never too old to do anything you desire. Bring it on.

# THANK YOU

I am beyond lucky to have so many beautiful people in my life. The past fifteen months have been the most challenging time for not only me, but for my loved ones.

The BCNA do such wonderful work supporting women and men diagnosed with breast cancer, the information they provide is so valuable in those early days and beyond. I am tremendously grateful to live here in Australia and have such fantastic resources available to me.

I am ever so grateful to the following people for their love and support:

Ray, Imogen and Trinity, my everything, always.

"The Marilyn's" (Janet, Kerry, Mel and Penny)
my girl power and chemo buddies.

Susan and Clare at White Space Yoga and Light Space Yoga.

The doctors, nurses and staff at Surrey Hills Health Matters,
big love to Sandra (aka the Nurse from heaven),
Dr. Marchant and Dr. Sitlington.

The nurses and staff at Epworth Box Hill Day Oncology
(Alwyn, Dianna, Sue, Jodie, Jo Jo, Dinah and Eddie)
you are all angels.

Mr. Millar, Dr Foo, Dr Wang and Dr Coxon.

To all the women (and two men!) on my BCNA
Tuscany Trek, you are awesome, big love to Franc, Kate,
Katrina, Monica and Ruth.

To my beautiful family who are always there for me.

The 4J's (Jane, John, Joanne and Joanie).

My Salco family.

To Andrew, for listening to me rave on for years.

Big love to Soraya and her mum!

Special thanks to my editor Heather
for her encouragement to a first time author.

Special appreciation to Michelle and her team
at Accentia Design for having faith in me.

To all my gorgeous friends who supported me
and to everyone who donated to my fundraising.

To Anna Blatman for her amazing artwork that
adorns my front cover.

To Siimon Reynolds, I'm glad your book found me.

To BCNA, what a truly remarkable and brilliant organisation. Special thanks to Paige for being my go-between .

Thank you to Inspired Adventures for an awesome trek and to Jenny for all her fundraising tips.

Melbourne writer, Jane Delahay shares with us a very personal journey with her first non-fiction book -
*The Leap Year*

Follow Jane on Facebook;
**Jane Delahay - Author**
or visit www.janedelahay.com

Jane's next book is underway and will be available in early 2018. It's called
*Four for the Road*

www.ingramcontent.com/pod-product-compliance
Lightning Source LLC
Chambersburg PA
CBHW071921290426
44110CB00013B/1431